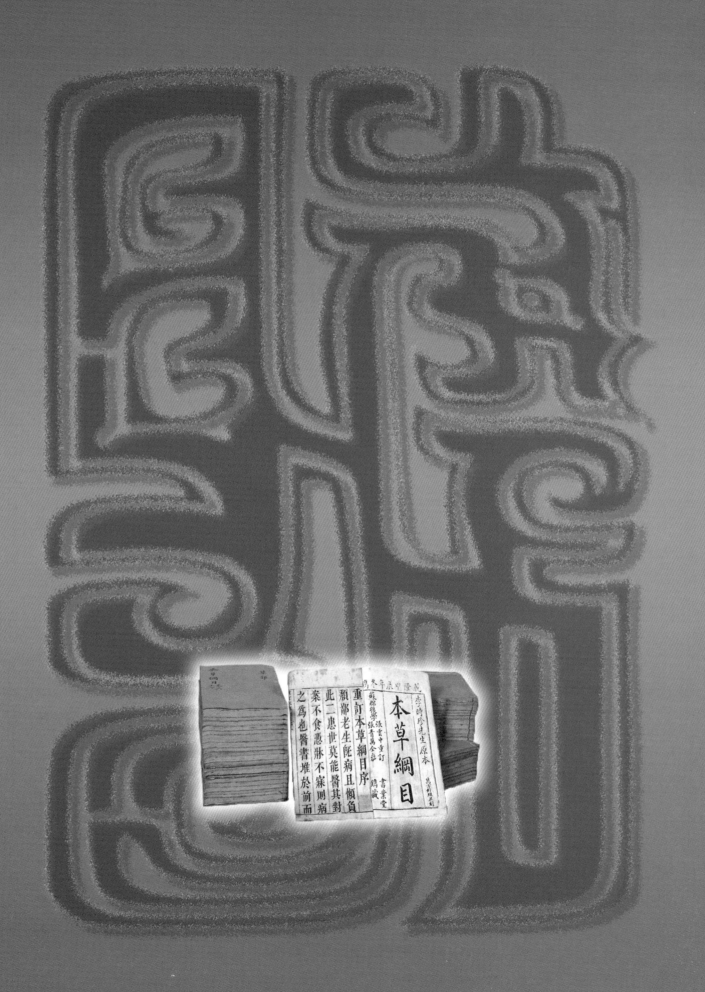

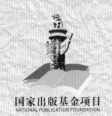

国家出版基金项目
NATIONAL PUBLICATION FOUNDATION

中华医药卫生

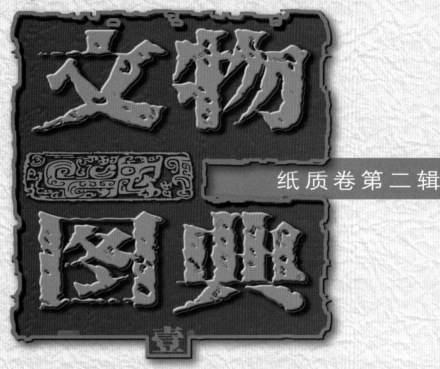

纸质卷第二辑

主　编　李经纬　梁　峻　刘学春

总主译　白永权

主　译　吉　乐

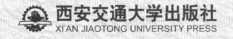

西安交通大学出版社
XI'AN JIAOTONG UNIVERSITY PRESS

图书在版编目 (CIP) 数据

中华医药卫生文物图典 .1. 纸质卷 . 第 2 辑 ./ 李经纬，
梁峻，刘学春主编 .— 西安：西安交通大学出版社，2016.12

ISBN 978-7-5605-7022-8

Ⅰ . ①中… Ⅱ . ①李… ②梁… ③刘… Ⅲ . ①中国医药学—
纸制品—文物—中国—图录 Ⅳ . ① R-092 ② K870.2

中国版本图书馆 CIP 数据核字（2015）第 013551 号

书　　名　中华医药卫生文物图典（一）纸质卷第二辑
主　　编　李经纬　梁　峻　刘学春
责任编辑　赵文娟

出版发行　西安交通大学出版社
　　　　　（西安市兴庆南路 10 号　邮政编码 710049）
网　　址　http://www.xjtupress.com
电　　话　（029）82668805　82668502（医学分社）
　　　　　（029）82668315（总编办）
传　　真　（029）82668280
印　　刷　中煤地西安地图制印有限公司

开　　本　889mm×1194mm　1/16　印张 35.5　字数　562 千字
版次印次　2017 年 12 月第 1 版　2017 年 12 月第 1 次印刷
书　　号　ISBN 978-7-5605-7022-8
定　　价　1080.00 元

读者购书、书店添货、如发现印装质量问题，请通过以下方式联系、调换。
订购热线：（029）82665248　（029）82665249
投稿热线：（029）82668805　（029）82668502
读者信箱：medpress@126.com

铭记感受历史

自信自重自强

书贺

中华医药卫生文物图典问世

陈可冀 谨题

二〇一七年肖月

陈可冀　中国科学院院士、国医大师

精修醫藥衛生文物

圖典功著當代

深究岐黃學術思想

淵源惠澤千秋

中華醫藥衛生文物圖典出版誌慶

丁酉孟秋 孫光榮 敬題於北京

孫光荣 国医大师

中華醫藥衛生文物圖典出版

彰顯中醫藥文化精神

體現中醫藥歷史價值

歲次丁酉夏 王琦

王琦 国医大师

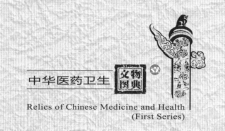

中华医药卫生

Relics of Chinese Medicine and Health
(First Series)

中华医药卫生文物图典（一）
丛书编撰委员会

主　编　李经纬　梁　峻　刘学春

副主编　廖　果　吴鸿洲　康兴军　和中浚　刘小斌　杨金生

　　　　　郑怀林　徐江雁　白建疆　黄　煌

编　委　李洪晓　梁永宣　王强虎　董树平　马　健　王　霞

　　　　　张雅宗　朱德明　包哈申　张建青　郑　蓉　庄乾竹

　　　　　李宏红　刘哲峰　王宏才　陈润东

总主译　白永权

主　译　陈向京　聂文信　范晓晖　温　睿　赵永生　杜彦龙

　　　　　吉　乐　李小棉　郭　梦　陈　曦

副主译（按姓氏音序排列）

　　　　　董艳云　姜雨孜　李建西　刘　慧　马　健　任宝磊

　　　　　任　萌　任　莹　王　颇　习通源　谢皖吉　徐素云

　　　　　许崇钰　许　梅　詹菊红　赵　菲　邹郝晶

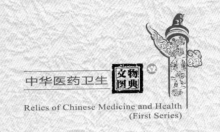

中华医药卫生 文物图典

Relics of Chinese Medicine and Health
(First Series)

本册编撰委员会

主　编	李经纬　梁　峻　刘学春
副主编	廖　果　吴鸿洲　康兴军　和中浚　刘小斌　杨金生
	郑怀林　徐江雁　白建疆　黄　煌
编　委	李洪晓　梁永宣　王强虎　董树平　马　健　王　霞
	张雅宗　朱德明　包哈申　张建青　郑　蓉　庄乾竹
	李宏红　刘哲峰　王宏才　陈润东

总主译	白永权
主　译	吉　乐
副主译	李小棉
译　者	王慧敏　迟征宇　张梦原　高　琛　王　媛
	牛笑语　吴耀均　黄　鋆　蒋新蕾　席　慧
	郭　宁　张继飞　刘雅恬

丛书策划委员会

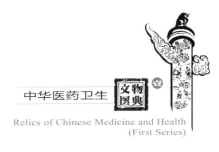

中华医药卫生 文物图典

Relics of Chinese Medicine and Health
(First Series)

序　言

　　探索天、地、人运动变化规律以及"气化物生"过程的相互关系，
是人类永恒的课题。宇宙不可逆，地球不可逆，人生不可逆业已成为共识。
天地造化形成自然，人类活动构成文化。文物既是文化的载体，又是物
化的历史，还是文明的见证。

　　追求健康长寿是人类共同的夙愿。中华民族之所以繁衍昌盛，健康
文化起了巨大的推动作用。由于古人谋求生存发展、应对环境变化产生
的智慧，大多反映在以医药卫生为核心的健康文化之中，所以，习总书
记说："中医药学是中国古代科学的瑰宝，也是打开中华文明宝库的钥匙"。

　　秉持文化大发展、大繁荣理念，中国中医科学院李经纬、梁峻等为
负责人的科研团队在完成科技部"国家重点医药卫生文物收集调研和保
护"课题获 2005 年度中华中医药学会科技二等奖基础上，又资鉴"夏
商周断代工程""中华文明探源工程"等相关考古成果，用有重要价值
的新出土文物置换原拍摄质量较差的文物，适当补充民族医药文物，共
精选收载 5000 余件。经西安交通大学出版社申报，《中华医药卫生文
物图典（一）》（以下简称《图典》）于 2013 年获得了国家出版基金
的资助，并经专业翻译团队翻译，使《图典》得以面世。

　　文物承载的信息多元丰富，发掘解读其中蕴藏的智慧并非易事。　医
药卫生文物更具有特殊性，除文物的一般属性外，还承载着传统医学发

展史迹与促进健康的信息。运用历史唯物主义观察发掘文物信息，善于从生活文物中领悟卫生信息，才能准确解读其功能，也才能诠释其在民生健康中的历史作用，收到以古鉴今之效果。"历史是现实的根源"，任何一个民族都不能割断历史，史料都包含在文化中。"文化是民族的血脉，是人民的精神家园"，文化繁荣才能实现中华民族的伟大复兴。值本《图典》付梓之际，用"梳理文化之脉，必获健康之果"作为序言并和作者、读者共勉！

中央文史研究馆馆员
中国工程院院士　王永炎
丁酉年仲夏

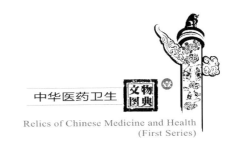

前 言

　　文化是相对自然的概念，是考古界常用词汇。文物是文化的重要组成部分，既是文明的物证，又是物化的历史。狭义医药卫生文物是疾病防治模式语境下的解读，而广义医药卫生文物则是躯体、心态、环境适应三维健康模式下的诠释。中华民族是 56 个民族组成的多元一体大家庭，中华医药卫生文物当然包括各民族的健康文化遗存。

　　天地造化如造山、板块漂移、气候变迁、生物起源进化等形成自然。气化物生莫贵于人，即整个生物进化的最高成果是人类自身。广义而言，人类生存思维留下的痕迹即物质财富和精神财富总和构成文化，其一般的物化形式是视觉感知的文物、文献、胜迹等。其中质变标志明晰的文化如文字、文物、城市、礼仪等可称作文明。从唯物史观视角观察，狭义文化即精神财富，尤其体现人类精、气、神状态的事项，其本质也具有特殊物质属性，如量子也具有波粒二相性，这种粒子也是物质，无非运动方式特殊而已。现代所谓可重复验证的"科学"，事实上也是从文化中分离出来的事项，因此也是一种特殊文化形式。追求健康长寿是人类共同的夙愿。中华民族之所以繁衍昌盛，是因为健康文化异彩纷呈。中华优秀传统医药文化之所以博大精深，是因为其原创思维博大、格物致知精深，所以，习总书记说："中医药学是中国古代科学的瑰宝，也是打开中华文明宝库的钥匙"。

文化既反映时代、地域、民族分布、生产资料来源、技术水平等信息，又反映人类认知水平和生存智慧。发掘解读文物、文献中蕴藏的健康知识和灵动智慧，首先是从事健康工作者的责任和义务。《易经》设有"观"卦，人类作为观察者，不仅要积极收藏展陈文物，而且要善于捕捉文物倾诉的信息，汲取养分，启迪思维，收到古为今用之效果。墨子三表法，首先一表即"本之于古者圣王之事"，也是强调古代史实的重要性。"历史是现实的根源"，现实是未来的基础。任何一个国家、地区、民族都不能割断历史、忽略基础，这个基础就是文化。"文化是民族的血脉，是人民的精神家园"。文化繁荣才能驱动各项事业发展，才能实现中华民族的伟大复兴。

人类从类人猿分化出来。"禄丰古猿禄丰种"是云南禄丰发现的类人猿化石，距今七八百万年。距今200万年前人类进入旧石器时代，直立行走，打制石器产生工具意识，管理火种，是所谓"燧人氏"时代。中国留存有更新世早、中期的元谋、蓝田、北京人等遗址。距今10万—5万年前，人类进入旧石器时代中期，即早期智人阶段，脑容量增加，和欧洲、非洲人种相比，原始蒙古人种颧骨前突等，是所谓"伏羲氏"时代。中国发现的马坝、长阳、丁村人等较典型。距今5万—1万年前，人类进入旧石器时代晚期，即晚期智人阶段，细石器、骨角器等遍布全国，山顶洞、柳江、资阳人等较典型。

中石器时代距今约1万年，是旧石器时代向新石器时代的短暂过渡期，弓箭发明，狗被驯化。河南灵井、陕西沙苑遗址等作为代表。距今1万—公元前2600年前后，人类进入新石器时代，磨光石器、烧制陶器，出现农业村落并饲养家畜，是所谓"神农氏"时代。公元前7000年以来，在甲、骨、陶、石等载体上出现契刻符号、七音阶骨笛乐器等，反映出人文气息趋浓。公元前6000—公元前3500年的老官台、裴李岗、河姆渡、马家浜、仰韶等文化遗址，彰显出先民围绕生存健康问题所做的各种努力。

公元前4800年以来，以关中、晋南、豫西为中心形成的仰韶文化，是中原史前文化的重要标志。以半坡、庙底沟类型为典型，自公元前3500年走向繁荣，属于锄耕粟黍稻兼营渔猎饲养猪鸡经济方式，彩陶尤其发达。公元前4400—公元前3300年，长江中游的大溪文化，薄胎彩陶和白陶发达。公元前4300—公元前2500年山东丰岛的大汶口文化，红陶为主。公元前3500年前后，辽东的红山文化原始宗教发展。公元前 3300 年以来，长江下游由河姆渡、马家浜文化衍续的良渚文化和陇西的马家窑文化、江淮间的薛家岗文化时趋发达。

公元前 2600—公元前 2000 年，黄河中下游龙山文化群形成，冶铸铜器，制作玉器，土坯、石灰、夯筑技术开始应用。公元前 2697 年，轩辕战败炎帝（有说其后裔）、蚩尤而为黄帝纪元元年。黄帝西巡访贤，"至岐见岐伯，引载而归，访于治道"。其引归地"溱洧襟带于前，梅泰环拱于后"，即今河南新密市古城寨。岐黄答问，构建《黄帝内经》健康知识体系，中华文明从关注民生健康起步。颛顼改革宗教，神职人员出现；帝喾修身节用，帝尧和合百国，舜同律度量衡，大禹疏导治水，中华民族不断繁衍昌盛。

公元前 2070 年，禹之子启以豫西晋南为中心建立夏王朝，二里头青铜文化为其特征，半地穴、窑洞、地面建筑并存。饮食卫生器具、酒器增多。朱砂安神作用在宫殿应用。公元前 1600 年，商灭夏。偃师商城设有铸铜作坊。公元前 1300 年，盘庚迁殷，使用甲骨文。武丁时期青铜浑铸、分铸并存。公元前 1056 年，相传周"文王被殷纣拘于羑里，演《周易》，成六十四卦"。公元前 1046 年，武王克商建周，定都镐京。青铜器始铸长篇铭文，周原发掘出微型甲骨文字。公元前 770 年，平王东迁。虢国铸铜柄铁剑。公元前 753 年，秦国设置史官。公元前 707 年出现蝗灾、公元前 613 年出现"哈雷彗星"，均被孔子载入《春秋》。公元前 221 年，秦始皇统一中国，多元一体民族大家庭形成，中华医药卫生文物异彩纷呈。

中国是治史大国，历来重视发展文化博物事业，1955 年成立卫生部中医研究院时就设置医史研究室，1982 年中国医史文献研究所成立时复建中国医史博物馆研究收藏展陈文物。2000—2003 年，经王永炎院士、姚乃礼院长等呼吁，科技部批准立项，由李经纬、梁峻为负责人的团队完成"国家重点医药卫生文物收集调研和保护"项目任务，受到科技部项目验收组专家的高度评价，获中华中医药学会科技进步二等奖。2013 年，在国家出版基金资助下，课题组对部分文物重新拍摄或必要置换、充实民族医药文物后，由西安交通大学出版社编辑、组聘国内一流翻译团队英译说明文字付梓，受到国家中医药博物馆筹备工作领导小组和办公室的高度重视。

"物以类聚"，《图典》主要依据文物质地、种类分为 9 卷，计有陶瓷，金属，纸质，竹木，玉石、织品及标本，壁画石刻及遗址，少数民族文物，其他，备考等卷。同卷下主要根据历史年代或小类分册设章。每卷下的历史时段不求统一。遵循上述规则将《图典》划分为 21 册，总计收载文物 5000 余件。对每件文物的描述，除质地、规格、馆藏等基本要素外，重点描述其在民生健康中的作用。对少数暂不明确的事项在括号中注明待考。对引自各博物馆的材料除在文物后列出馆藏外，还在书后再次统一列出馆名或参考书目，以充分尊重其馆藏权，也同时维护本典作者的引用权。

21 世纪，围绕人类健康的生命科学将飞速发展，但科学离不开文化，文化离不开文物。发掘文物承载的信息为现实服务，谨引用横渠先生四言之两语："为天地立心，为生民立命"，既作为编撰本《图典》之宗旨，也是我们践行国家"一带一路"倡议的具体努力。希冀通过本《图典》的出版发行，教育国人，提振中华民族精神；走向世界，为人类健康事业贡献力量。

李经纬　梁峻　刘学春

2017 年 6 月于北京

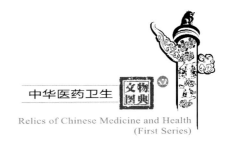

中华医药卫生 文物图典
Relics of Chinese Medicine and Health
(First Series)

目 录

1

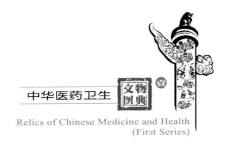

Contents

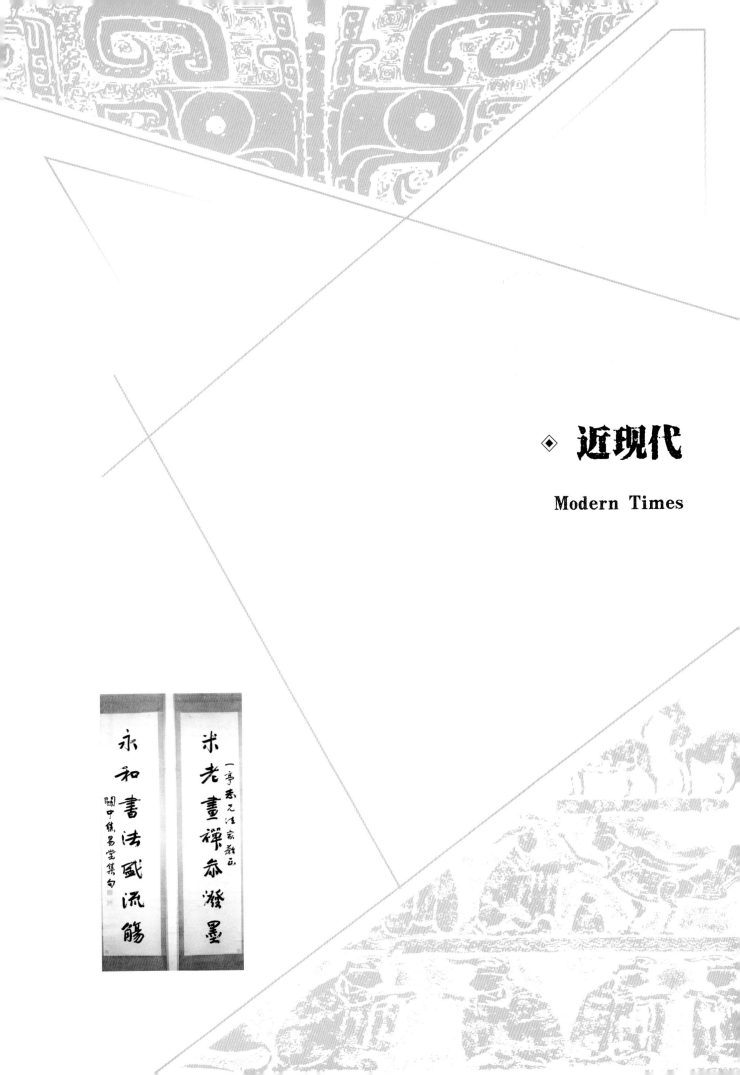

◇ **近现代**

Modern Times

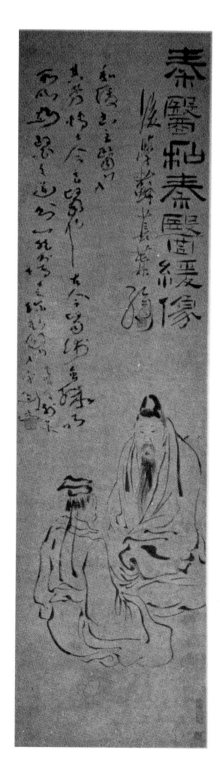

医和、医缓画像

清

长 134 厘米，宽 30 厘米

Portrait of Doctor He and Doctor Huan

Qing Dynasty

Length 134 cm/ Width 30 cm

医和、医缓，春秋时期秦国名医。此画像系
清代岭南派画家苏长春所绘。曹仲英捐献。

上海中医药博物馆藏

He and Huan were famous doctors of Qin State
in the Spring and Autumn Periods. This portrait
was painted by Su Changchun, a Lingnan-style
painter in the Qing Dynasty. It was donated by
Cao Zhongying.

Preserved in Shanghai Museum of Traditional
Chinese Medicine

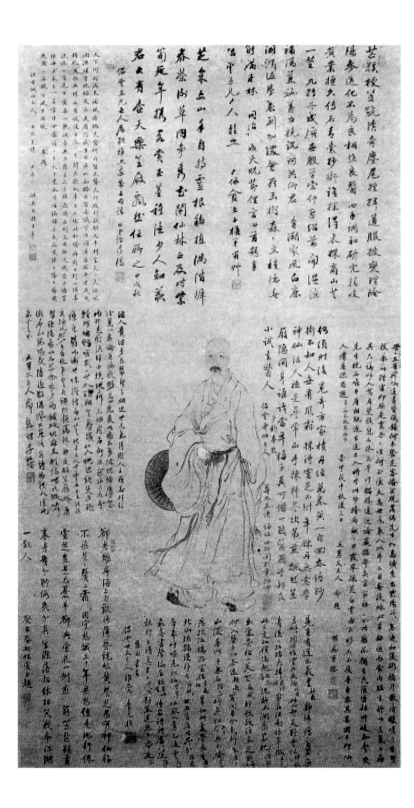

朱侣云画像

清

长 97 厘米，宽 53.5 厘米

清·闵彤章绘。朱氏为清代医生。

上海中医药博物馆藏

Portrait of Zhu Lüyun

Qing Dynasty

Length 97 cm/ Width 53.5 cm

The portrait was painted by Min Tongzhang in the Qing Dynasty. Zhu was a doctor in the Qing Dynasty.

Preserved in Shanghai Museum of Traditional Chinese Medicine

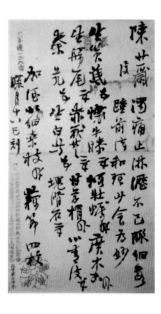

何鸿舫处方

清

整体：92 厘米 ×39 厘米

局部：22 厘米 ×13 厘米

何鸿舫为清代名医，用药好选黄芪、地黄、党参、白术等，所用印章外圆内方为钱币形，方孔有"读书不官乃为医"；另一印章梅花形，每一花瓣占一字，曰："重古梅花卢"。何氏擅文，与当时公卿多应酬，盛名由来于此不无关系。

广东中医药博物馆藏

Prescription from He Hongfang

Qing Dynasty

Holistic: 92 cm×39 cm

Part: 22cm×13cm

He Hongfang was a famous doctor in the Qing Dynasty preferring to use Astragalus, Rehmannia, Dangshen and Atractylodes, etc. Within the cylindrical side of the coin-shaped seal is a square hole in which are characters "Du Shu Bu Guan Nai Wei Yi", which literally means that if educated people are not willing to be officials, they can be doctors. As to another plum-shaped seal, five characters "Zhong Gu Mei Hua Lu" are on plum's petals one by one. He was proficient at literary works and had social engagement with aristocracy, which brought part of his fame.

Preserved in Guangdong Chinese Medicine Museum

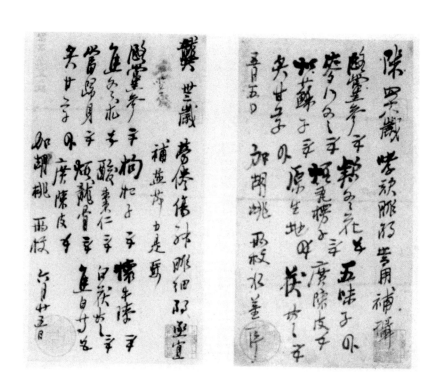

何鸿舫处方

清

长 23 厘米，宽 10.2 厘米

Prescription of He Hongfang

Qing Dyansty

Length 23 cm/ Width 10.2 cm

何鸿舫 (1821—1889)，清代医学家，原名昌治，后改长治，一字补之，晚号横泖病鸿，上海青浦人。世为医，已历 24 代，曾续其父所著《医人史传》《重固三何医案》。此为其手书处方笺。

上海中医药博物馆藏

He Hongfang (1821–1889) was a doctor in the Qing Dynasty. His original name was Changzhi, which then was changed into Changzhi. He was from Qingpu (now Shanghai City). Born in a family with 24 generations engaged in medical practice, he continued his father's medical works *Yi Ren Shi Zhuan* (Biography of Doctors) and *Zhong Gu San He Yi An* (Medical Cases of Zhonggu Sanhe). This is his handwritten prescription.
Preserved in Shanghai Museum of Traditional Chinese Medicine

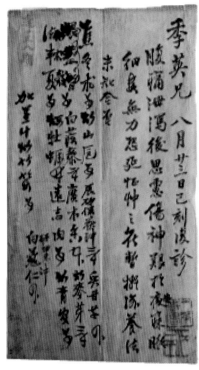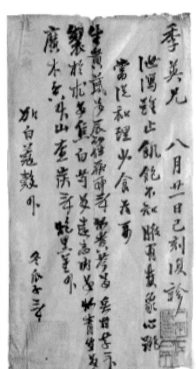

何鸿舫方笺

清

长 24.2 厘米，宽 12.9 厘米

Prescriptions Written by He Hongfang

Qing Dynasty

Length 24.2 cm/ Width 12.9 cm

清代医家何鸿舫真迹方笺。此为季英兄之泄
泻复诊医案二则。

江苏省中医药博物馆藏

These are the authentic prescriptions from
Doctor He Hongfang in the Qing Dynasty. They
were made for Ji Yingxiong's subsequent visits
for diarrhea.
Preserved in Jiangsu Museum of Traditional
Chinese Medicine

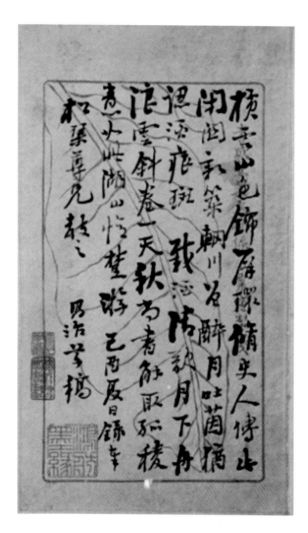

清代名医何鸿舫诗稿手迹

清

9 厘米 ×5 厘米

Handwriting of He Hongfang's Poem

Qing Dynasty

9 cm×5 cm

何鸿舫为清代名医，医术高超，并精于书法，墨数行只字，人成宝之，竟有乔装病人而为获其墨宝。

　　　　广东中医药博物馆藏

He Hongfang was a famous doctor in the Qing Dynasty as well as an artist in calligraphy. People treasured his calligraphic works very much even though there were just a few characters. Someone even pretended tohe a patient in order to get his calligraphy.

Preserved in Guangdong Chinese Medicine Museum

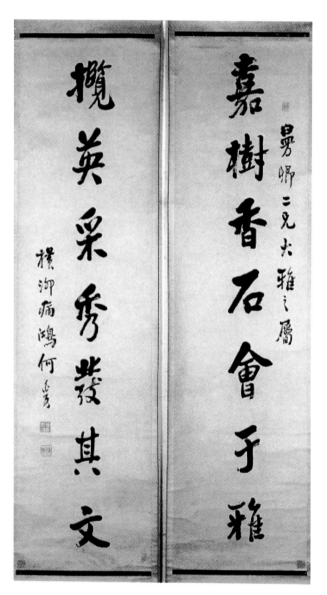

何鸿舫书联

清

长 150 厘米，宽 39.5 厘米

Couplets Written By He Hongfang

Qing Dynasty

Length 150 cm/ Width 39.5 cm

何鸿舫，清代江南名医，同治、光绪年间以医学和书法闻名于沪上。其字竖拔浑厚，力透纸背。此楹联内容为"嘉树香石会于雅，榄英采秀发其文"。

上海中医药博物馆藏

He Hongfang was a famous doctor in the regions south of the Yangtze River in the Qing Dynasty. During the reign of Emperor Tongzhi and Guangxu, he became prestigious because of his medical science and calligraphy. His calligraphy is straight and powerful, and seems to be able to penetrate the paper. The couplet transcribes one of his poetic sentences (14 Chinese characters describing the relationship between the beauty of nature and that of literature).
Preserved in Shanghai Museum of Traditional Chinese Medicine

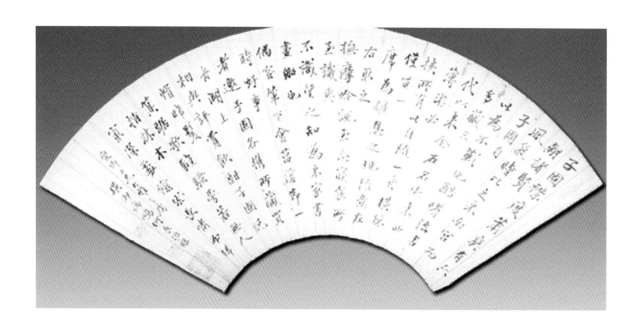

何鸿舫书扇

清

长 51.5 厘米，高 17 厘米

何鸿舫书法学颜平原、李北海等诸家，雄健浑厚。
其既精医术，又工书法，时人获其处方珍若拱璧。

上海中医药博物馆藏

Calligraphy on a Fan by He Hongfang

Qing Dynasty

Length 51.5 cm/ Height 17 cm

He Hongfang's handwriting, with the simple and
vigorous style, imitated calligraphy works of
famous calligraphers such as Yan Pingyuan and Li
Beihai. He was proficient in both medical science
and calligraphy; therefore, people of his time
regarded his prescriptions as treasures.

Preserved in Shanghai Museum of Traditional
Chinese Medicine

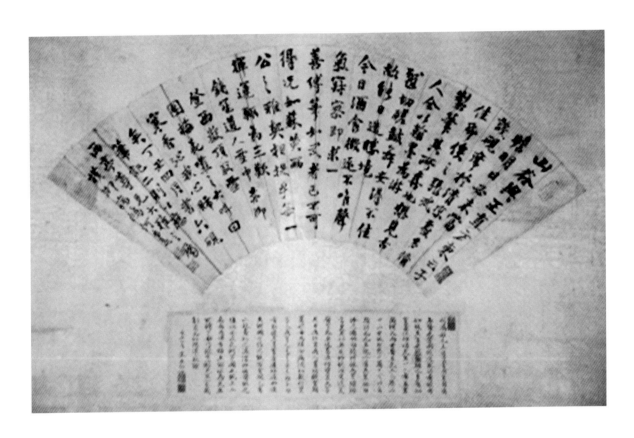

何鸿舫手书扇页挂图

清

58 厘米 ×39 厘米

何鸿舫为清代名医，用药好选黄芪、地黄、党参、白术等，并精于书法，墨数行只字，人成宝之，竟有乔装病人而为获其墨宝。

广东中医药博物馆藏

Calligraphy on a Wall Fan by He Hongfang

Qing Dynasty

58 cm×39 cm

He Hongfang was a famous doctor in the Qing Dynasty preferring to use Astragalus, Rehmannia, Dangshen and Atractylodes, etc. He was also a calligrapher. People treasured his calligraphic works very much even though there were just a few words. Someone even pretended tohe a patient in order to get his calligraphy.

Preserved in Guangdong Chinese Medicine Museum

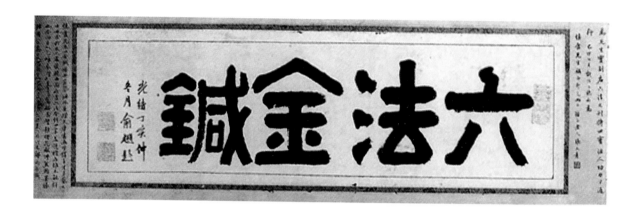

俞樾题"六法金针"横额

清

长 96.5 厘米，宽 30 厘米

Banner "Liu Fa Jin Zhen" by Yu Yue

Qing Dynasty

Length 96.5 cm/ Width 30 cm

俞樾 (1821—1907)，字荫甫，号曲园，浙江
德清人。道光三十年 (1850) 进士，清末儒学
大师，重要医学著述有《废医记》《枕上三
字诀》《内经辨言》。

上海中医药博物馆藏

Yu Yue (1821–1907, courtesy name Yinfu,
assumed name Quyuan, from Deqing County of
Zhejiang Province), was a famous scholar and
calligrapher in the Qing Dynasty. He passed
the imperial examination in 1850 (the 30th year
of Emperor Daoguang's reign) and became a
Confucian master during the late Qing Dynasty.
His significant medical books include "Fei Yi
Lun" (*On Abolishing the Traditional Chinese
Medicine*), "Zhen Shang San Zi Jue" (*Three-
word Tactic for A Good Sleep*), and "Nei Jing
Bian Yan" (Collation on the Internal Canon of
Medicine).
Preserved in Shanghai Museum of Traditional
Chinese Medicine

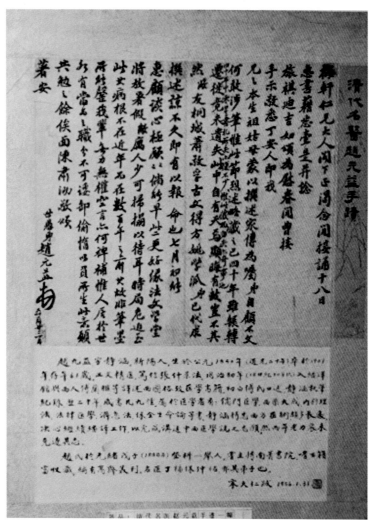

清代名医赵元益手迹

清

36 厘米 ×25 厘米

Handwriting of Famous Doctor Zhao Yuanyi in Qing Dynasty

Qing Dynasty

36 cm×25 cm

赵元益，字静涵，新阳人，生于 1840 年，卒于 1902 年。工文精医，笃信仲景之学。同治初年入翻译馆，与西方人傅兰雅等译西国格致医学书籍，成书九种，其中属于医学的有：《儒门医学》《西药大成》《内科理法》《法律医学》等。

广东中医药博物馆藏

Zhao Yuanyi (1840–1902, courtesy name Jinghan), was born in Xinyang County. He was good at writing and medical science, with strong belief in the theory of Zhang Zhongjing (one of the most famous Chinese physicians in the history). In the early years of the reign of Emperor Tongzhi, Zhao Yuanyi entered the Translation House and translated with John Fryer western medical books of nine categories, such as *Ru Men Yi Xue*, *Xi Yao Da Cheng*, *Nei Ke Li Fa*, and *Fa Lv Yi Xue* (these books are about western medicine, pharmacy, internal medicine and forensic medicine) .
Preserved in Guangdong Chinese Medicine Museum

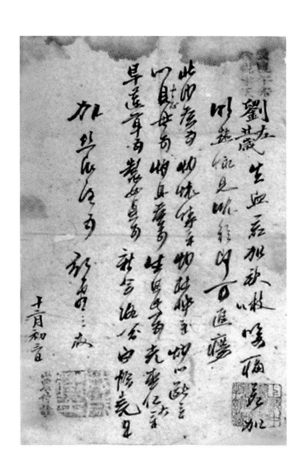

陈莲舫处方

清

23.6 厘米 ×13 厘米

Prescription Written by Chen Lianfang

Qing Dynasty

23.6 cm×13 cm

长方形，为中医处方，由白纸黑墨书成，是陈莲舫给 21 岁的刘先生开的处方。陈莲舫（1837—1914)，名秉钧，清著名医家，上海青浦人，世业医。1912 年创设上海医会，先后五次进宫为光绪帝医疾，封三品官，弟子甚众，门人董韵笙所辑《陈莲舫医案秘钞》可窥其医术端倪。保存基本完好，纸张泛黄，有水浸迹。1963 年入藏。

中华医学会 / 上海中医药大学医史博物馆藏

This rectangular prescription, which was written by Chen Lianfang with black ink on the white paper, was made for 21-year-old Mr. Liu. Chen Lianfang (1837–1914, given name Bingjun) was a famous doctor from a family with generations of doctors in Qingpu County of Shanghai in the Qing Dynasty. Chen Lianfang established Shanghai Medical Association in the year 1912 and entered the emperor's palace for five times to make diagnosis and give treatment for Emperor Guangxu. Being offered the third-rank official position in imperial China, he had many disciples, and his medical skills were displayed in *"Chen Lianfang Yi An Mi Chao"* (a medical book contains Chen Lianfang's diagnosis and treatment of diseases) written by Dong Yunsheng, one of Chen Lianfang's apprentices. This prescription is preserved in basically good condition with yellowing and water logging papers. It was collected in 1963.

Preserved in Chinese Medical Association/Museum of Chinese Medicine History, Shanghai University of Traditional Chinese Medicine

陈莲舫处方

清

23.6 厘米 × 13 厘米

长方形，为中医处方，由白纸黑墨书成，是陈莲舫给 49 岁的高女士开的处方。保存基本完好，纸张泛黄，有水浸迹。1963 年入藏。

中华医学会 / 上海中医药大学医史博物馆藏

Prescription Written by Chen Lianfang

Qing Dynasty

23.6 cm×13 cm

This rectangular traditional Chinese medical prescription, written with black ink on white paper, was given to 49-year-old Ms. Gao by Chen Lianfang. This prescription is preserved in basically good condition with yellow discoloration and water logging stains on the paper. It was collected in 1963.

Preserved in Chinese Medical Association/ Museum of Chinese Medicine, Shanghai University of Traditional Chinese Medicine

陈莲舫处方

清

23.5 厘米 ×12.8 厘米

长方形，为中医处方，由白纸黑墨书成，是陈莲舫给 38 岁的沈女士开的处方。保存基本完好，纸张泛黄，有水浸迹。1963 年入藏。

中华医学会 / 上海中医药大学医史博物馆藏

Prescription Written by Chen Lianfang

Qing Dynasty

23.5 cm×12.8 cm

This rectangular traditional Chinese medical prescription, written with black ink on white paper, was given to 38-year-old Ms. Shen by Chen Lianfang. This prescription is preserved in basically good condition with yellowing and water logging papers. It was collected in 1963.

Preserved in Chinese Medical Association/ Museum of Chinese Medicine, Shanghai University of Traditional Chinese Medicine

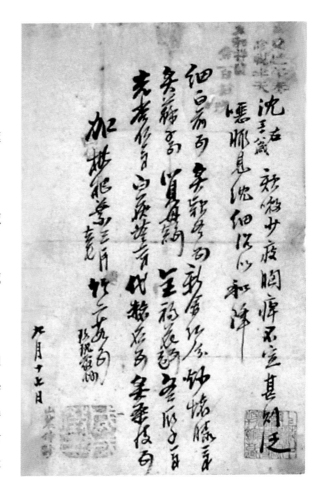

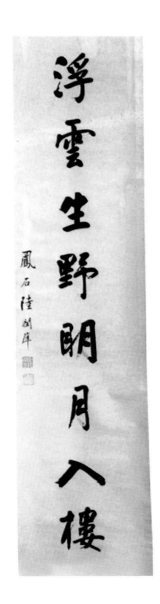
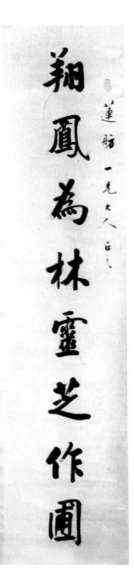

陆润庠书八言联

清

长 165 厘米，宽 42 厘米

此为其书赠晚清医学家陈莲舫之对联。内容为：

"翔凤为木棂芝作图，浮云生野明月入楼"。

上海中医药博物馆藏

Couplets Written by Lu Runyang

Qing Dynasty

Length 165 cm/ Width 42 cm

This pair of couplets was written by Lu Runyang (an official in the late Qing Dynasty) as a gift to Chen Lianfang, a famous medical scientist. It writes 16 Chinese characters describing the natural scene.

Preserved in Shanghai Museum of Traditional Chinese Medicine

"柳致和堂"包装纸

清

长 21.2 厘米 ，宽 18.4 厘米

晚清名医柳宝诒药堂所用。纸上印有朱字"柳致和堂大房精制各种丸散"，地址为"江阴周庄镇东街，三阳门东首"。

江苏省中医药博物馆藏

Wrapping Paper of "Liu Zhi He Tang" Drugstore

Qing Dynasty

Length 21.2 cm/ Width 18.4 cm

This wrapping paper was used by the drugstore of Liu Baoyi, a famous doctor in the late Qing Dynasty. There are 26 red Chinese characters on the paper, which means that the "Liu Zhi He Tang" drugstore has all kinds of refined and useful pill and powder, and the address is San Yang Men Dong Shou, East Street, Zhouzhuang Town of Jiangyin County.

Preserved in Jiangsu Museum of Traditional Chinese Medicine

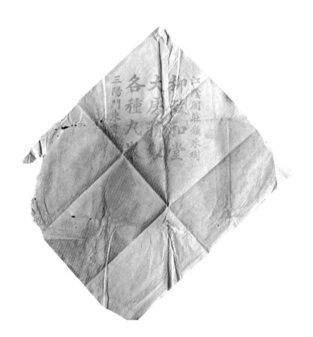

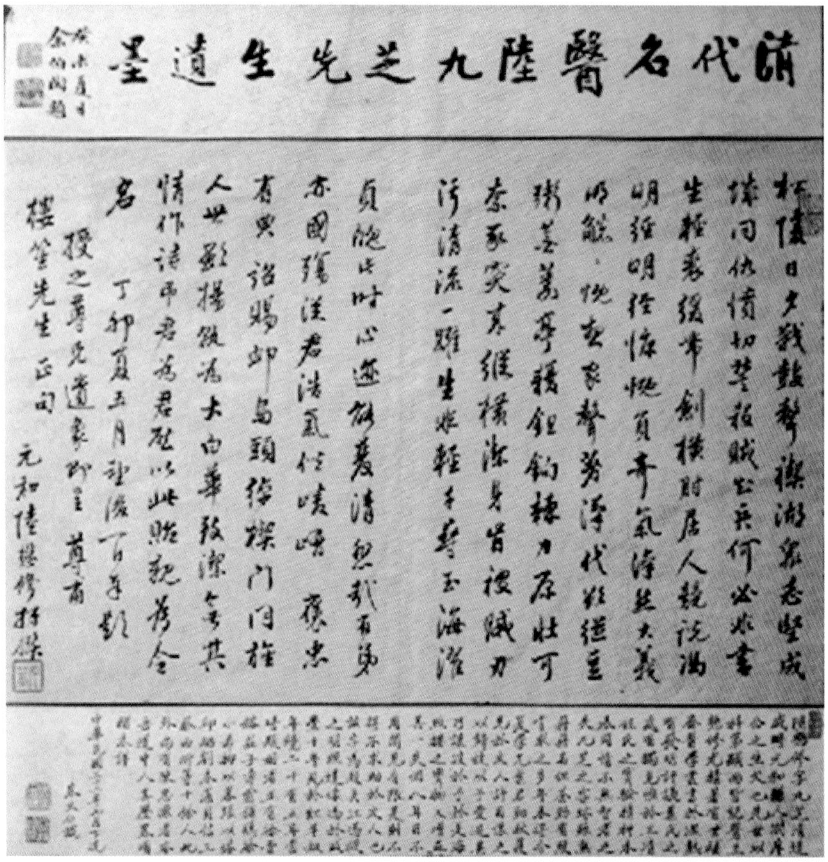

清代名医陆九芝先生墨迹

清

44 厘米 ×44 厘米

Handwriting of Famous Doctor Lu Jiuzhi

Qing Dynasty

44 cm×44 cm

陆懋修，字九芝，清道光咸丰时人，先祖以科举及弟，而通医，至懋修尤精医学，著有《世补斋医书》。对温病学热病有发明，对叶天士的评论有独特见解。其字苍劲有致。

广东中医药博物馆藏

Lu Maoxiu (courtesy name Jiuzhi) was a famous doctor during the reigns of Emperor Daoguang and Xianfeng in the Qing Dynasty. His ancestors had passed the imperial examination and were proficient in medical science, while Liu Maoxiu was especially expert in medical science and has written *"Shi Bu Zhai Yi Shu"* (a series of medical books). He created new treatments on epidemic febrile disease and pyreticosis, and had unique understanding about the ideas of Ye Tianshi (a famous doctor who lived in the Qing Dynasty, one of the most famous doctors who treated epidemic febrile disease). His calligraphy is vigorous and forceful.

Preserved in Guangdong Chinese Medicine Museum

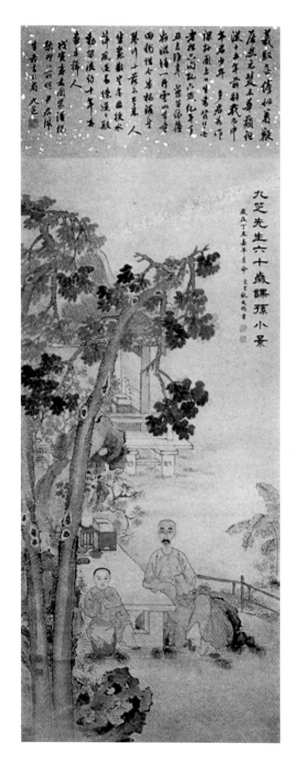

九芝先生 60 岁课孙小景图

清

长 130 厘米，宽 50 厘米

Painting of 60-Year-old Lu Jiuzhi Teaching Grandson (Small Picture)

Qing Dynasty

Length 130 cm/ Width 50 cm

陆懋修，字九芝，苏州元和县人，生于嘉庆戊寅（1818），卒于光绪年间。先世以儒著称，皆通医。其中年始肆力于医，活人无数，学精《内经》、运气、治宗仲景之法，著有《世补斋医书之集》《不榭枋》《伤寒论阳明病释》《仲景方汇录》等。

上海中医药博物馆藏

Lu Maoxiu (courtesy name Jiuzhi, from Yuanhe County of Suzhou City), was born in 1818 (the 23rd year of Emperor Jiaqing's reign) and died during the reign of Emperor Guangxu in the Qing Dynasty. His ancestors were known for Confucianism and they were all proficient in medical science. Lu devoted himself to medical science and saved countless people, mastering the Internal Canon of Medicine, Yun Qi (directing one's strength to a specific part of the body through concentration) and methods of medical sage Zhang Zhongjing. He wrote many medical books such as *Shi Bu Zhai Yi Xue Wen Ji* (a series of medical books), *Bu Xie Fang* (a collection of over 30 effective prescriptions), *Shang Han Lun Yang Ming Bing Shi* (a medical book of explanations of the Treatise on Febrile and Miscellaneous Diseases), and *Zhong Jing Fang Hui Lu* (a collection of Zhang Zhongjing's prescriptions).

Preserved in Shanghai Museum of Traditional Chinese Medicine

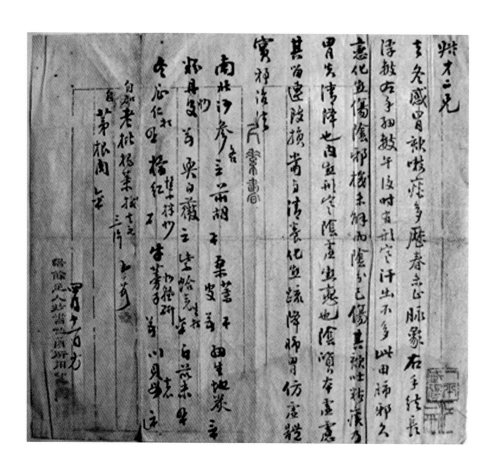

柳宝诒方笺

清

长 26.5 厘米，宽 24 厘米

Prescription Written by Liu Baoyi

Qing Dynasty

Length 26.5 cm/ Width 24 cm

清代名医柳宝诒真迹方笺。柳宝诒（1842—1901），字谷孙，号冠群，江苏江阴县（今江阴市）周庄镇东街人。清光绪十六年（1890）开设"柳致和堂"药店，1894年又在江阴城东开设"柳致和堂"分店。著有《素问说意》《惜余医活》《柳选四家医案》《惜余医案》《柳致和堂丸散膏丹释义》《疟痢逢源》《温热逢源》等。

江苏省中医药博物馆藏

This prescription is the authentic work of Liu Baoyi's handwriting. Liu Baoyi (1842-1901, courtesy name Gusun, assumed name Guanqun) came from East Street, Zhouzhuang Town, Jiangyin County of Jiangsu Province (now Jiangyin City). He opened the "Liu Zhi He Tang" drugstore in 1890 (the 16th year of Emperor Guangxu's reign), and a branch store at the east of Jiangyin City in 1894. He had written many books including *Su Wen Shuo Yi* (a book of questions and explanations related to medical science), *Xi Yu Yi Hua* (a book about medical remarks), *Liu Xuan Si Jia Yi An* (a medical book of case studies of four famous doctors in Qing Dynasty), *Xi Yu Yi An* (a book of medical case studies), *Liu Zhi He Tang Wan San Gao Dan Shi Yi* (an instruction book for drugs produced by Liu Zhi He Tang), *Nue Li Feng Yuan* (a medical book of malaria), and *Wen Re Feng Yuan* (a medical book of epidemic febrile diseases).

Preserved in Jiangsu Museum of Traditional Chinese Medicine

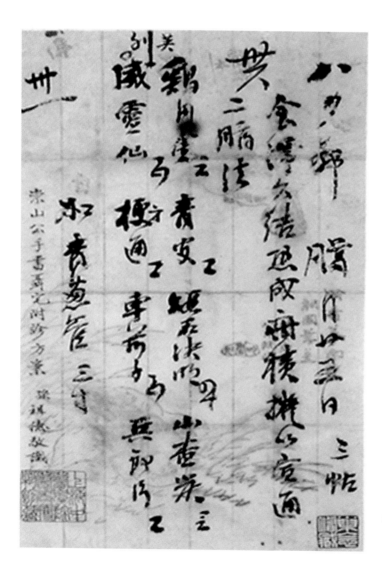

巢崇山处方

清

23.7 厘米 ×12.3 厘米

Prescription Written by Chao Chongshan

Qing Dynasty

23.7 cm ×12.3 cm

长方形，为处方。该处方用巢氏专用处方纸写成，是巢崇山所开治疗食滞疳积的处方，有后辈"巢念修藏"章。方末印有"崇山公手书聂宅附诊方案"等字样。巢崇山（1843－1909），武进孟河人，清医家，著有《玉壶仙馆外科医案》《巢崇山医案》《千金珍秘》。保存基本完好。1960年入藏。

中华医学会／上海中医药大学医史博物馆藏

This rectangular prescription was written by Chao Chongshan on his special note-paper to treat dyspepsia and infantile malnutrition, and there is a seal of his descendant with the characters of "Chao Nian Xiu Cang" (preserved by Chao Nian Xiu). At the end of this prescription are printed characters meaning that Mr. Chao Chongshan wrote the diagnosis and medical treatment for Nies' family. Chao Chongshan (1843–1909), born in Menghe Town of Wujin County, was a medical scientist in the Qing Dynasty. He was the author of *Yu Hu Xian Guan Wai Ke Yi An* (a book of clinical case study), *Chao Chong Shan Yi An* (Medical Case Study of Chao Chongshan) and *Qian Jin Zhen Mi* (precious and secret prescriptions). This prescription was collected in 1960 and is kept in basically good condition. Preserved in Chinese Medical Association/ Museum of Chinese Medicine, Shanghai University of Traditional Chinese Medicine

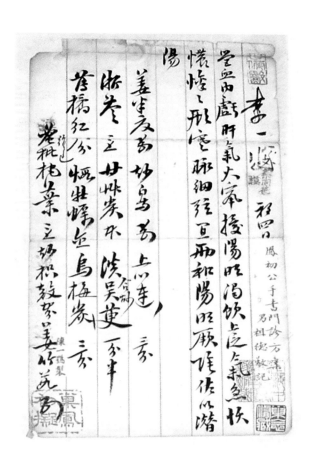

巢凤初处方

清

23.7 厘米 ×12.5 厘米

Prescription Written by Chao Fengchu

Qing Dynasty

23.7 cm×12.5 cm

长方形，为处方，用巢氏专用处方纸写成，是巢凤初为李氏所开处方，有"巢凤初拟"押记，上方钤"世儒医"章，下有后辈"巢念修藏"章。巢凤初，武进孟河人，清医家，擅内科，精刀圭之术。其父为巢崇山。保存基本完好。

中华医学会 / 上海中医药大学医史博物馆藏

This rectangular prescription, written on Chaos' special notepaper. It was given by Chao Fengchu for patient Li, and there is a seal with characters of "Chao Feng Chu Ni" (prescribed by Chao Fengchu). On the upward side, there is a seal with characters of "Shi Ru Yi" (scholar-physician for generations); on the bottom, his descendant's seal with the characters of "Chao Nian Xiu Cang" (preserved by Chao Nianxiu) is printed. Chao Fengchu, born in Menghe Town of Wujin County, was a medical scientist in the Qing Dynasty who was proficient in internal medicine and medical surgery. His father was Chao Chongshan. This prescription is kept in basically good condition.

Preserved in Chinese Medical Association/ Museum of Chinese Medicine, Shanghai University of Traditional Chinese Medicine

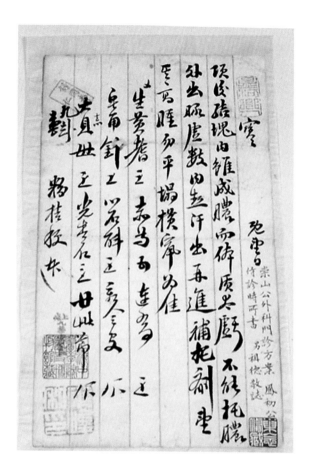

巢崇山处方

清

23.7 厘米 ×12.3 厘米

Prescription Written by Chao Chongshan

Qing Dynasty

23.7 cm×12.3 cm

长方形，为处方。该处方用巢氏专用处方纸写成，是巢崇山
所开治疗食滞疳积的处方，有后辈"巢念修藏"章。方末印
有"崇山公手书聂宅附诊方案"等字样。其子巢凤初擅内科，
精刀圭之术。保存基本完好。1960 年入藏。

中华医学会 / 上海中医药大学医史博物馆藏

This rectangular prescription was written by Chao Chongshan
on his special note-paper to treat dyspepsia and infantile
malnutrition. There is a seal of his descendant with the characters
of "Chao Nian Xiu Cang" (preserved by Chao Nian Xiu). At the
end of this prescription are printed characters of meaning that Mr.
Chao Chongshan wrote the diagnosis and medical treatment for
Nie's family). His son Chao Fengchu was proficient in internal
medicine and medical surgery. This prescription was collected in
1960 and is kept in basically good condition.

Preserved in Chinese Medical Association/ Museum of Chinese
Medicine, Shanghai University of Traditional Chinese Medicine

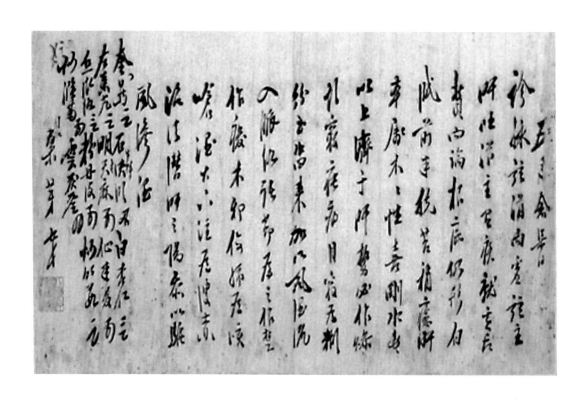

金子久亲笔脉案

清

处方：长 51.3 厘米，宽 24.1 厘米

册页：37.8 厘米 ×28.8 厘米

Jin Zijiu's Handwritten Medical Record

Qing Dynasty

Prescription: Length 51.3 cm/ Width 24.1 cm

Album:37.8 cm×28.8 cm

册页，为处方。据《桐乡县志》载，金子久（1870—1921），名有恒，祖籍武林，后徙大麻，桐乡名医。幼从父习医，后自学成名。性敦厚，谦逊好学，恒手不释卷，尤赞赏喻昌之《寓意草》，得力于叶氏《临证指南》。其弟子著《问松堂医案》《金子久医案》可窥其学术端倪。已裱成册页，保存基本完好。1957 年入藏。

中华医学会 / 上海中医药大学医史博物馆藏

This album is a prescription. According to *Tong Xiang Xian Zhi* (A local chronicle of Tongxiang County), Jin Zijiu (1870–1921), whose given name is You Heng, was from Wulin County (now Hangzhou City), and later moved to Dama Town. He was a well-known doctor in Tongxiang County. Jin Zijiu had been studying traditional Chinese Medicine from his father since childhood, and then he became a famous doctor by self-study. As an honest, humble and intelligent person, he appreciated Yu Chang's *Yu Yi Cao* (a medical book), and was inspired by *Lin Zheng Zhi Nan* (Case Report for Clinical Practice) by Ye. From the books like *Wen Song Tang Yi An* (Medical Cases of WensongTang) and *Jin Zi Jiu Yi An* (Medical Cases of Jin Zijiu) written by his students, we can know his academic achievement. This prescription has been mounted into an album. It was collected in 1957 and is well preserved.

Preserved in Chinese Medical Association/ Museum of Chinese Medicine, Shanghai University of Traditional Chinese Medicine

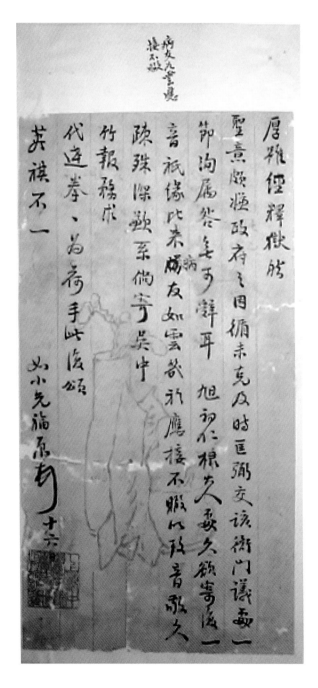

薛福辰笔札

清

长 22.8 厘米，宽 12.5 厘米

Writing by Xue Fuchen

Qing Dynasty

Length 22.8 cm/ Width 12.5 cm

笔札，为信函。该藏行书写就，行文流畅自如。薛福辰，字瘦吟，又字抚屏，江苏吴县人，清代医学家。曾与马文植同被荐治慈禧太后疾。著有《医学发微》《临证一得》等书。此为其手书札记，其中有入宫诊病的记载。保存完好。1959 年入藏。

中华医学会 / 上海中医药大学医史博物馆藏

This writing material is a letter, and was written in running script. The handwriting is smooth and free. Xue Chenfu, courtesy name Shouyin or Fuping, born in Wuxian County, Jiangsu Province, was a medical scientist in the Qing Dynasty. Once he was recommended with Ma Wenzhi to treat disease for Empress Dowager Ci Xi. He had written some medical books, such as *Yi Xue Fa Wei* and *Lin Zheng Yi De*. This letter was written by himself and recorded that he made a diagnosis in the imperial palace. It is well preserved, and was collected in 1959.

Preserved in Chinese Medical Association/ Museum of Chinese Medicine, Shanghai University of Traditional Chinese Medicine

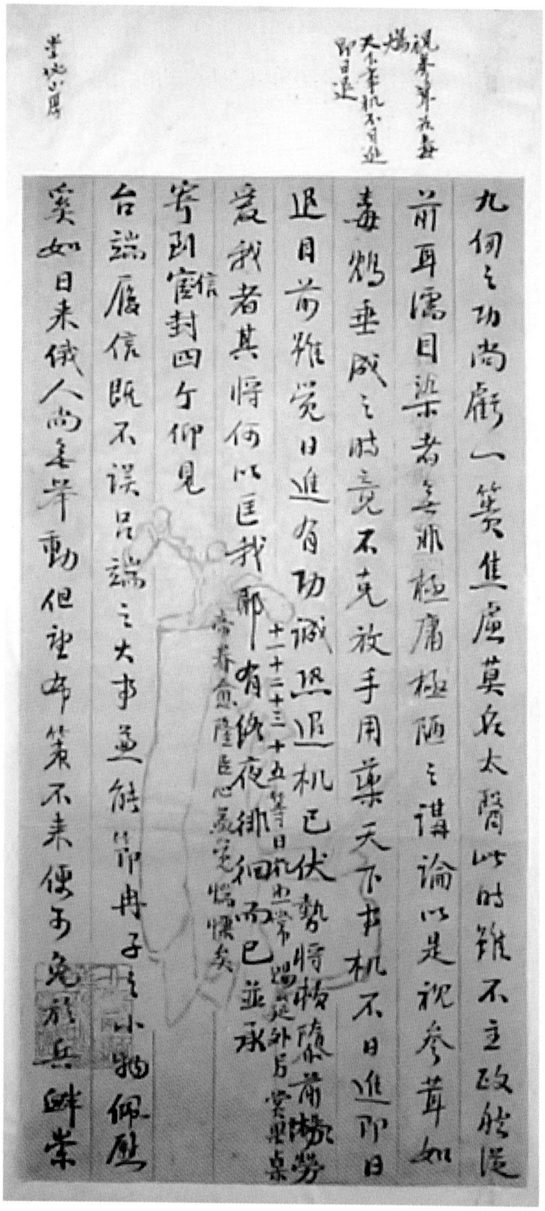

薛福辰笔札

清

长 18 厘米，宽 6.8 厘米

Writing by Xue Fuchen

Qing Dynasty

Length 18 cm/ Width 6.8 cm

笔札，为信函。该藏行书写就，行文流畅自如。此为其手书札记，其中有入宫诊病的记载。保存完好。1959 年入藏。

中华医学会 / 上海中医药大学医史博物馆藏

This writing material is a letter, and was written in running script. The handwriting is smooth and free. It recorded that he made a diagnosis in the imperial palace. It is well preserved, and was collected in 1959.

Preserved in Chinese Medical Association/Museum of Chinese Medicine, Shanghai University of Traditional Chinese Medicine

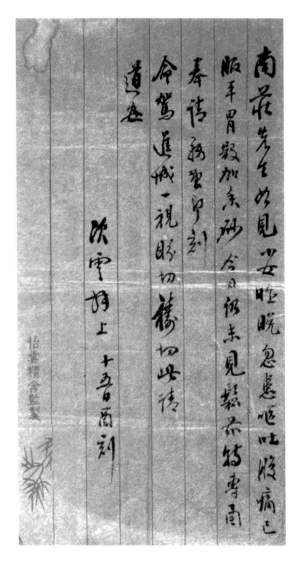

求医函

清

长 24 厘米，宽 13 厘米

Letter for Seeking a Doctor

Qing Dynasty

Length 24 cm/ Width 13 cm

该藏在清末四川西昌名医吴兰庄《医圣合璧》手稿中发现。函中述"小女昨晚忽患呕吐腹痛，已服平胃散加香砂，今日仍未见松，兹特专函奉请，务望即到"。

　　成都中医药大学中医药传统文化博物馆藏

It was discovered in a medical manuscript *Yi Sheng He Bi* by Wu Lanzhuang who was a famous doctor in Xichang City, Sichuan Province in the Qing Dynasty. This letter recorded that "My daughter suddenly fell ill last night with vomit and stomache, and has took Pingwei Powder and Xiangsha (a kind of medicine in treating dyspepsia). However, she was not better today. So, I wrote this letter to ask for a doctor. Please save my daughter if you see the letter".

Preserved in Museum of Traditional Chinese Medicine Culture, Chengdu University of Traditional Chinese Medicine

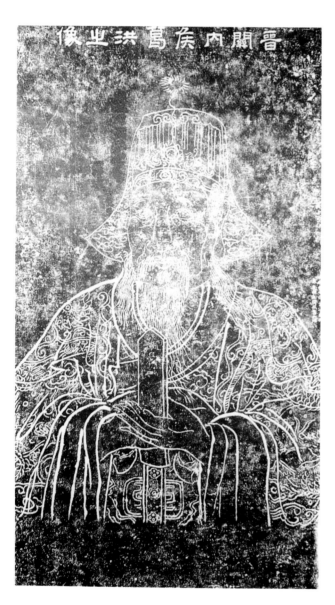

葛洪像拓片

清

长 120.2 厘米，宽 58 厘米

Rubbing of the Carved Image of Ge Hong

Qing Dynasty

Length 120.2 cm/ Width 58 cm

此为杭州西湖葛岭碑刻拓片。葛洪（284—
364），字稚川，自号抱朴子，丹阳句容（今江苏）
人。东晋时期道教理论家、医学家、炼丹术士，
编撰《肘后救卒方》《抱朴子》《金匮药方》等
著作，对古代化学、医学都有杰出贡献。

上海中医药博物馆藏

This is a rubbing of a stone tablet in Geling,
West Lake of Hangzhou. Ge Hong (281-364)
was born in Jurong, Danyang (now in Jiangsu
Province). His style name, also known as courtesy
name, was Zhichuan, and he gave himself a
pseudonym Baopuzi. He was a Taoist theorist,
physician, and alchemist in the Eastern Jin Dynasty.
With many prominent works including *Zhou
Hou Jiu Zu Fang* (Handbook of Prescriptions for
Emergencies), *Bao Fu Zi* (valuable material for the
research on Taoism), and *Jin Kui Yao Fang* (Golden
Prescriptions), he made great contributions to
ancient chemistry and medicine.
Preserved in Shanghai Museum of Traditional
Chinese Medicine

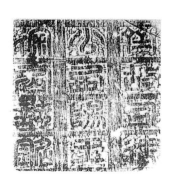

徐之才墓志拓片

清

长 55 厘米，宽 30 厘米

徐之才，南北朝北齐医家，出身世医家庭，少聪慧，年十三召为太学生，以医名驰于北地。其撰有《药对》《小儿方》等书，均佚。

上海中医药博物馆藏

Rubbing of Xu Zhicai's Epitaph

Qing Dynasty

Length 55 cm/ Width 30 cm

Xu Zhicai, a doctor of Northern Qi Dynasty during the Northern and Southern Dynasties, was born in a medical family. With great talent he was admitted by the Imperial College at age of 13 and was very famous in northern part of China for his medical skills. He wrote several medical books such as *Yao Dui* (a book about dings) and *Xiao Er Fang* (a book about pediatrics), but they were all lost.

Preserved in Shanghai Museum of Traditional Chinese Medicine

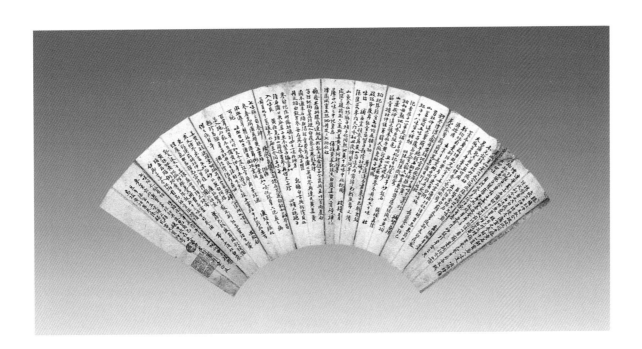

药方书扇

清

长 51 厘米

古代医生常将众多药方抄写于扇面上，以便诊治疾病时随时检索。

上海中医药博物馆藏

Fan-Shaped Book for Prescription

Qing Dynasty

Length 51cm

Doctors in ancient China used to transcribe many prescriptions on fans, so that they could check them through when necessary.

Preserved in Shanghai Museum of Traditional Chinese Medicine

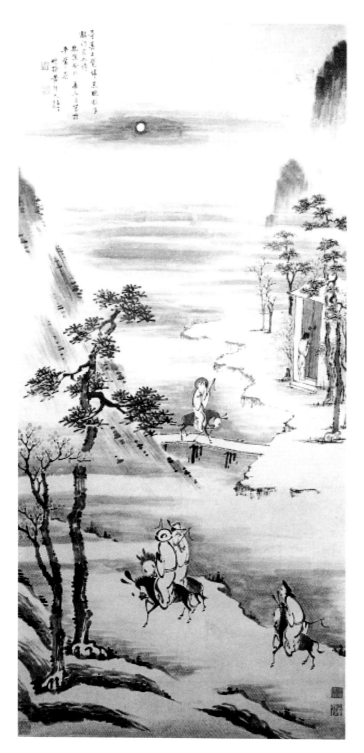

黄叔元山水图轴

清

长 13 厘米，宽 6 厘米

黄氏字云山，号草桥，江苏长洲草桥人。
通医，以小儿科知名；又精绘画，尤擅
画驴。

上海中医药博物馆藏

Scroll of Landscape Painting by Huang Shuyuan

Qing Dynasty

Length 130 cm/ Width 60 cm

Huang Shuyuan (courtesy name Yunshan, pseudonym name Caoqiao) was born in Caoqiao Town, Changzhou City, Jiangsu Province. He was a general doctor and was famous for pediatrics. He was also proficient in painting, especially drawing donkey.

Preserved in Shanghai Museum of Traditional Chinese Medicine

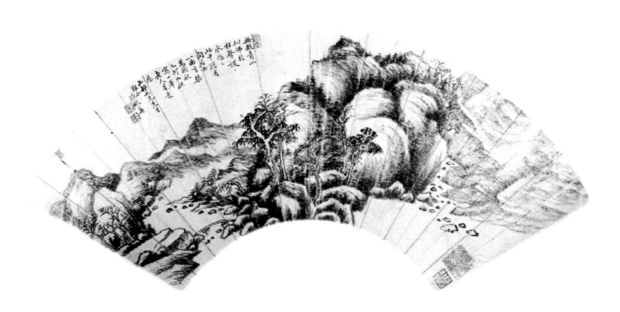

张查山山水图扇面

清

长 49 厘米，高 16.8 厘米

张查山，名璿，清代名医，著名山水画家。

上海中医药博物馆藏

Landscape Painting on Fan by Zhang Chashan

Qing Dynasty

Length 49 cm/ Height 16.8 cm

Zhang Chashan, also known with another name Xuan, was a renowned doctor and prominent landscape painter in the Qing Dynasty.

Preserved in Shanghai Museum of Traditional Chinese Medicine

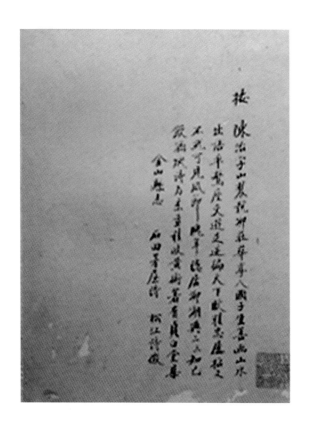 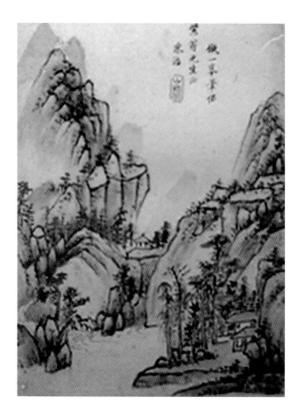

陈治山水画

清

26 厘米 ×20 厘米

Landscape Painting by Chen Zhi

Qing Dynasty

26 cm×20 cm

册页，为艺术品。该藏是陈治送给紫翁先生的山水画，已装裱成册页，有陈治落款和山农钤记。另附后人按，介绍陈治生平简历。陈治，字山农，华亭人，清代医家，平生好游，足迹遍及天下。精忠闻世，喜丹青，工诗文，精医术，著有《证治大还》《外台秘典》《贞白堂稿》等。保存基本完好。1958 年入藏。

中华医学会 / 上海中医药大学医史博物馆藏

This album is an artwork. This is a landscape painting which Chen Zhi gave to Mr. Ziweng, and has been mounted in album. It was signed with seals "Chen Zhi" and "Shan Nong Qian Ji" and another seal by descendants, which makes a brief introduction about Chen Zhi, whose courtesy name was Shannong, and who was born in Huating County. He was a doctor in the Qing Dynasty, and was fond of sightseeing and travelled around the country. He was famous for the loyalty to his country, and he loved painting and poems. He was also skillful at treating diseases, and wrote some medical books, such as *Zheng Zhi Da Huan*, *Wai Tai Mi Dian* and *Zhen Bai Tang Gao*. It was collected in 1958 and is well preserved.

Preserved in Chinese Medical Association/ Museum of Chinese Medicine, Shanghai University of Traditional Chinese Medicine

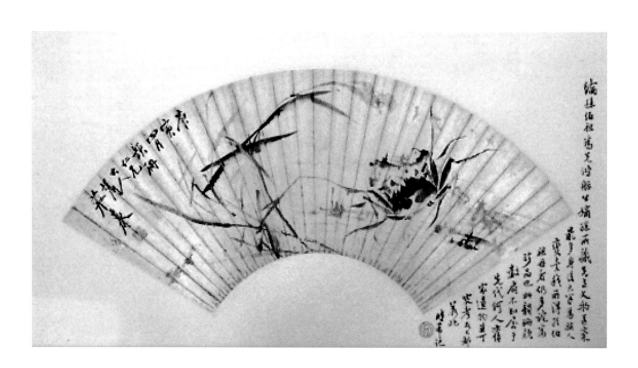

庄农芦蟹泥金扇面

清

扇面上宽 53 厘米，下宽 21.8 厘米，高 18.4 厘米
镜片，为艺术品，系清人庄农所作，韵珊款。镜
片右端有何时希题记。已装裱成镜片，保存基本
完好。1991 年入藏。

中华医学会 / 上海中医药大学医史博物馆藏

Painting of Crabs on Gold-flecked Fan by Zhuang Nong

Qing Dynasty

Upper Part of Fan 53 cm/ Lower Part of Fan 21.8 cm/ Height 18.4 cm

This painting was drawn by Zhuang Nong in the Qing Dynasty with the style of "Yun Shan". There is an inscription by He Shixi on the right of the fan. It is well preserved. It was collected in 1991.

Preserved in Chinese Medical Association/ Museum of Chinese Medicine, Shanghai University of Traditional Chinese Medicine

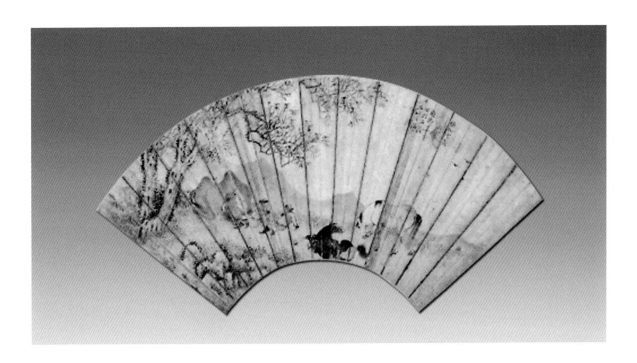

姜福卿人物走兽扇面

清

扇面上宽 48 厘米，下宽 20.8 厘米，高 17.1 厘米
镜片，为艺术品，系清人姜福卿所作。扇面右上
题款为"橅松雪翁"、"福卿姜画□于左花右竹
之居"，并钤白文"福"，朱文"卿"两印。已
装裱成镜片，保存基本完好。1991 年入藏。

　　　中华医学会 / 上海中医药大学医史博物馆藏

Painting of People and Animals on Fan by Jiang Fuqing

Qing Dynasty

Upper Part of Fan 48 cm/ Lower Part of Fan
20.8 cm/ Height 17.1 cm

This painting was drawn by Jiang Fuqing in the
Qing Dynasty. There are inscriptions of "Mo Song
Xue Weng" (old man with pines and snow) and
"Fuqing Jiang drew it at his home with flowers and
bamboo" on the upper right of the fan. The painter
affixed an intaglio seal "Fu" and a relief seal "Qing".
This fan has been framed. It is well-preserved. It
was collected in 1991.

Preserved in Chinese Medical Association/ Museum
of Chinese Medicine, Shanghai University of
Traditional Chinese Medicine

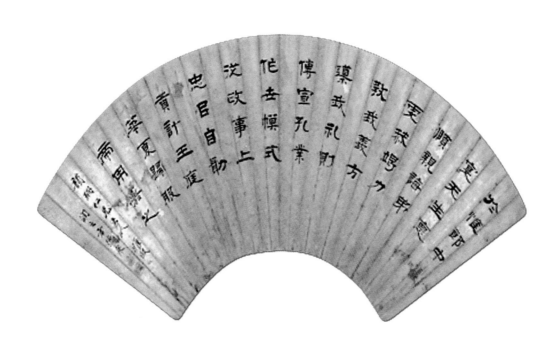

方德泉隶书泥精扇面

清

扇面：上宽 52.8 厘米，下宽 22.2 厘米，高 18.1 厘米

册页：长 61.5 厘米，宽 32.9 厘米

Clerical Script Calligraphy on Gold-flecked Fan by Fang Dequan

Qing Dynasty

Fan: Upper Width 52.8 cm / Lower Width 22.2 cm / Height 18.1 cm

Album: Length 61.5 cm / Width 32.9 cm

扇状，是艺术品，为清代方德泉所作。扇面为金黄色，

方德泉亲笔隶书 42 字，题赠韵珊，落款"润云方德泉"

并朱印记两方。已装裱成镜片，保存基本完好。1991 年

入藏。

中华医学会 / 上海中医药大学医史博物馆藏

It was made by Fang Dequan in the Qing Dynasty. This fan
is colored in gold. There are 42 characters written by Fang
Dequan in clerical script with an inscription "Yun Shan".
The calligrapher affixed two relief seals after the signiture
"Run Yun Fang De Quan". This fan has been framed. It is
well preserved. It was collected in 1991.

Preserved in Chinese Medical Association/ Museum of
Chinese Medicine, Shanghai University of Traditional
Chinese Medicine

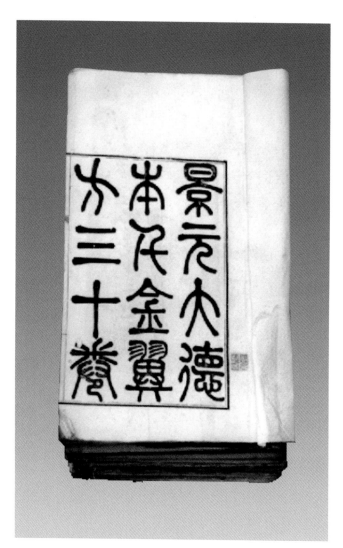

《千金翼方》一套十册

清

长31厘米，宽18.1厘米，重1 900克

Qian Jin Yi Fang (10 Chapters)

Qing Dynasty

Length 31cm/ Width 18.1 cm/ Wight 1,900 g

该藏为清光绪年影印宋体。《千金翼方》为唐代著名医学家孙思邈所著，与《千金要方》合称《千金方》，代表唐代先进的医学水平，在《千金要方》的基础上进一步论述了各种病证、诊治，并记载了其对药物学的研究成就。全书辑录800多种药物，并吸收许多外来药物，专列两卷记载对《伤寒杂病论》的研究。

广东中医药博物馆藏

The book shown in the picture is a copy of the Song Dynasty edition during the reign of Emperor Guangxu in the Qing Dynasty. *Qian Jin Yi Fang* was literally translated as the *Supplement to the Thousand Golden Remedies*. The book shown in the picture was a block-printed edition during the reign of Emperor Guangxu. *Qian Jin Yi Fang* was written by a famous doctor Sun Simiao in the Tang Dynasty. It along with *Qian Jin Yao Fang* (The Precious Formulas Worth a Thousand Gold) are called *Qian Jin Fang* (Essential Formulas Worth a Thousand Pieces of Gold), which represented the advanced medical level in the Tang Dynasty. *Qian Jin Yi Fang*, on the basis of the *Qian Jin Yao Fang*, further discussed various symptoms of diseases and relating diagnosis and treatment. *Qian Jin Yi Fang* also recorded the achievement of the study of medicines and listed more than 800 medicines including many foreign medicines. It had two special chapters that recorded the study of the book named *Shang Han Za Bing Lun* (Treatise on Typhia and Miscellaneous Illnesses).
Preserved in Guangdong Chinese Medicine Museum

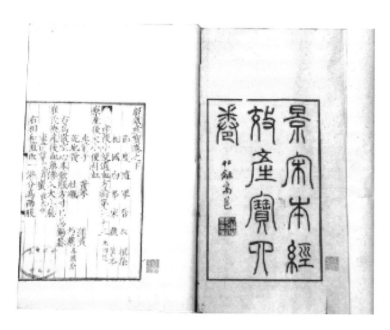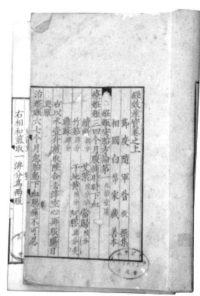

《经效产宝》一套两册

清

长 29.4 厘米，宽 17.5 厘米，重 375 克

Jing Xiao Chan Bao (2 Volumes)

Qing Dynasty

Length 29.4 cm/ Width 17.5 cm/ Weight 375 g

该藏为清光绪年影印宋体，唐代昝殷著，是我国现存第一部妇产科专著，收录了有关经闭、带上、坐月、难产、产后诸疾等备验药方，论及妊娠杂病、难产诸病及多种生产病，并介绍了治疗方法，许多论述至今仍有指导意义，如难产"内宜用药，外宜用法"。

广东中医药博物馆藏

The book shown in the picture is a copy of the Song Dynasty edition during the reign of Emperor Guangxu in the Qing Dynasty. The *Jing Xiao Chan Bao* was written by Zan Yin in the Tang Dynasty, which was the earliest treatise on gynaecology and obstetrics among the remaining medical works in China. It listed the prescriptions for amenorrhea, leukorrhea, confinement in childbirth, difficult labour and disorders after childbirth. It also discussed multiple obstetrical disorders and related miscellaneous illnesses as well as the corresponding treatments. Many theories in the *Jing xiao Chan Bao* can still serve as a guideline, such as the principle that difficult labour should be dealt with a combination method by strengthening nutrition of the pregnant woman as well as exerting the surgical operation to help the baby.

Preserved in Guangdong Chinese Medicine Museum

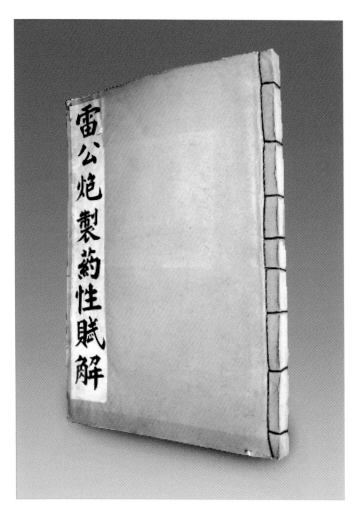

《雷公炮制药性赋解》

清

47.3 厘米 ×32 厘米

Lei Gong Pao Zhi Yao Xing Fu Jie

Qing Dynasty

47.3 cm×32 cm

线装书，医籍。其全称《增补珍珠囊雷公炮制药性赋解》，金人东垣李杲（字明之）编辑。该藏为清代线装精抄本。现藏有缺页。保存基本完整，纸张泛黄，局部磨损有蛀孔。1959 年入藏。

中华医学会 / 上海中医药大学医史博物馆藏

The book was assembled by traditional thread binding. The whole name of it was the *Zeng Bu Zhen Zhu Nang Lei Gong Pao Zhi Yao Xing Fu Jie* (a book about medicine). The book was compiled by Li Gao from Dongyuan in the Jin Dynasty. The collection shown in the picture was the Qing Dynasty edition. Some of the pages of the book were lost. The book is basically well preserved with yellow discolouration and partial abrasion and wormhole. It was collected in 1959.

Preserved in Chinese Medical Association/ Museum of Chinese Medicine, Shanghai University of Traditional Chinese Medicine

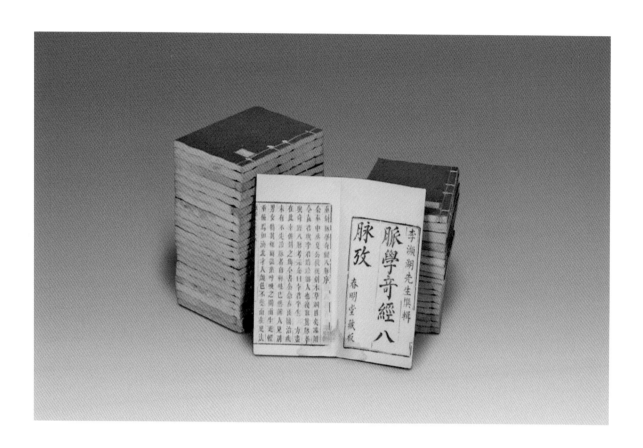

《本草纲目》

清

26.7 厘米 ×18.4 厘米

Ben Cao Gang Mu

Qing Dynasty

26.7cm ×18.4 cm

书本形，医籍。《本草纲目》(附《濒湖脉学考》
《奇经八脉考》《本草万方针线》)，明代
医家李时珍著。该藏本为春明堂版，清同治
壬申年（1872）重镌，芥子园苏郡后学张云
中重订，张青万仝纂，全书共40册，雕版线装。
保存基本完整，纸张泛黄，局部磨损。

中华医学会 / 上海中医药大学医史博物馆藏

Ben Cao Gang Mu (Compendium of Materia
Medica) was written by Li Shizhen in the Ming
Dynasty. The books are a collected edition by
"Chun Ming Tang" (the name of a publishing
house), which were made during the reign of
Emperor Tongzhi (1872), revised by Zhang
Yunzhong and edited by Zhang Qingwan.
The medical works had 40 volumes and were
assembled by traditional thread binding.
The books are basically well preserved, with
yellowing paper and partial abrasion.
Preserved in Chinese Medical Association/
Museum of Chinese Medicine, Shanghai
University of Traditional Chinese Medicine

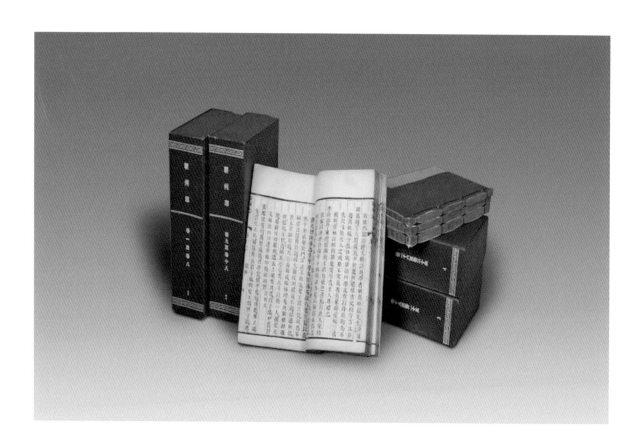

蕲州志

清

25.2 厘米 ×15.2 厘米

Qizhou Annals

Qing Dynasty

25.2 cm×15.2 cm

书本形，史籍。《蕲州志》为蕲州知事岭西封蔚礽纂修。全书共 18 册。清光绪八年季冬麟山书院重刊本。保存基本完整，纸张泛黄，局部磨损。

中华医学会 / 上海中医药大学医史博物馆藏

The books were written by magistrate Feng Weiqi in Qizhou (now in Huanggang City, Hubei Province). The books shown in the picture have 18 volumes, which are a reprinted edition by "Ji Dong Lin Shan Shuyuan" (the name of an academy of classical learning) in the 8th year of reign of Emperor Guangxu. The books are basically well preserved with yellowing paper and partial abrasion.

Preserved in Chinese Medical Association/ Museum of Chinese Medicine, Shanghai University of Traditional Chinese Medicine

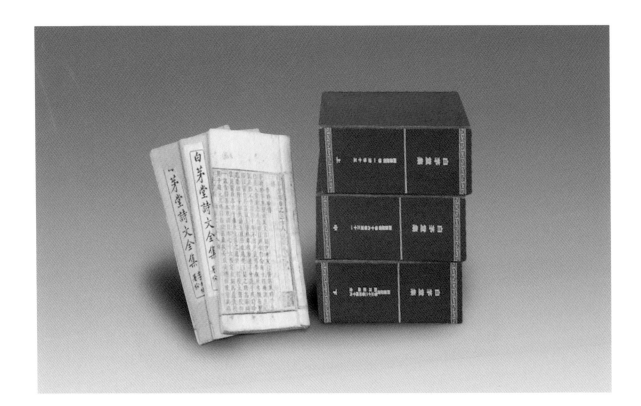

《白茅堂诗文全集》

清

25.1 厘米 ×15.8 厘米

Bai Mao Tang Shi Wen Quan Ji

Qing Dynasty

25.1 cm×15.8 cm

书本形，史籍。《白茅堂诗文全集》为明人李士彬署检，金州喻成龙作序，第三十八卷载李时珍传。全书共 20 册，雕版线装。保存基本完整，纸张泛黄，局部损。

中华医学会 / 上海中医药大学医史博物馆藏

Bai Mao Tang Shi Wen Quan Ji was translated as "complete works of poetic prose of Bai Mao Tang". As a historical work, its content was arranged and inspected by Li Shibin and its preface was written by Yu Chenglong from Jinzhou (now in Dalian City, Liaoning Province). The 38th volume of the book was biography of Li Shizhen. The book has twenty volumes and was assembled with traditional tread binding method. The book is basically well preserved with yellowing paper and partial abrasion.

Preserved in Chinese Medical Association/ Museum of Chinese Medicine, Shanghai University of Traditional Chinese Medicine

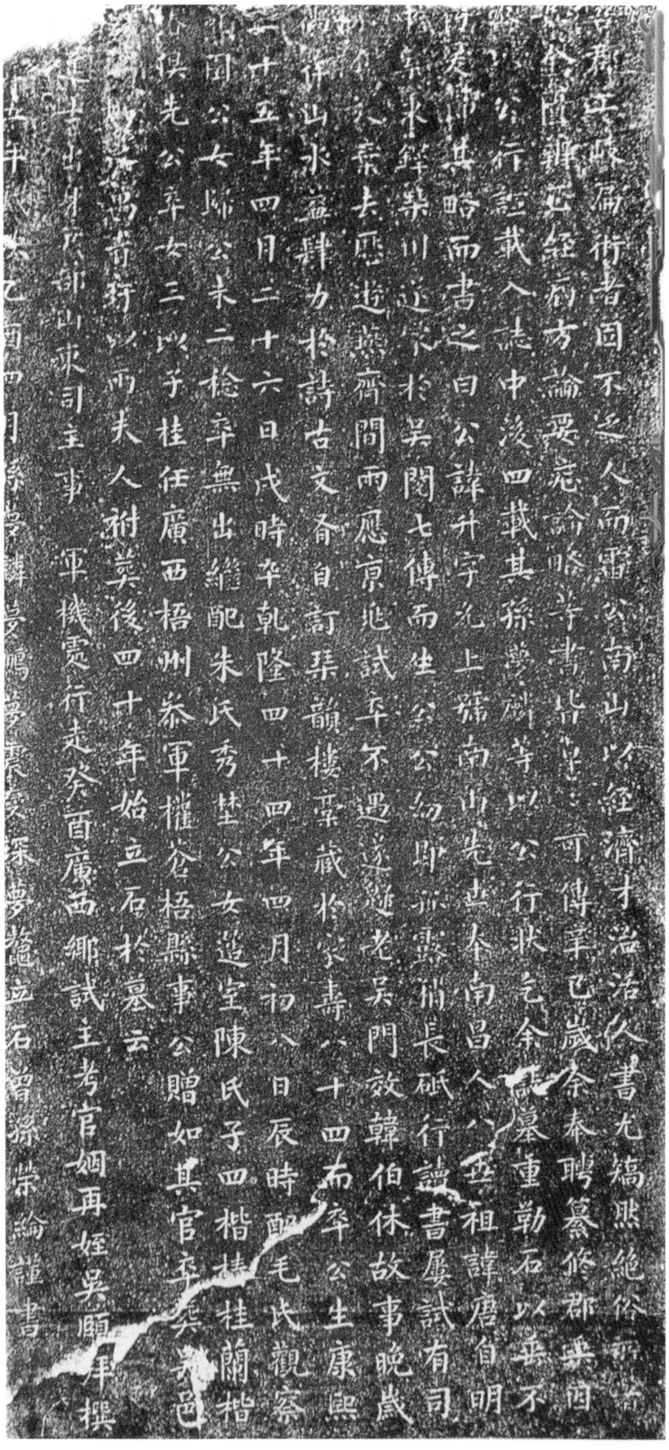

雷允上墓志拓片

清

长 69 厘米，宽 33.5 厘米

Rubbing of Lei Yunshang 's Tombstone

Qing Dynasty

Length 69 cm/ Width 33.5 cm

雷允上，名大升，号南山，江苏吴县人。清乾隆元年（1736）起以医行世，尤精配制丸、散、膏、丹，开有"雷允上药铺"，今存并享名国内外。

上海中医药博物馆藏

Lei Yunshang (courtesy name Da Sheng, pseudonym Nan Shan) was born in Wu Xian County in Jiangsu Province. From the 1st year of the reign of Emperor Qianlong (1736), Lei Yunshang started practicing medicine. He specialized in formulating pills, powder, ointment and pellet. He had opened a drug store named "Lei Yunshang Yao Pu", which still remains today and makes a name in home and abroad.

Preserved in Shanghai Museum of Traditional Chinese Medicine

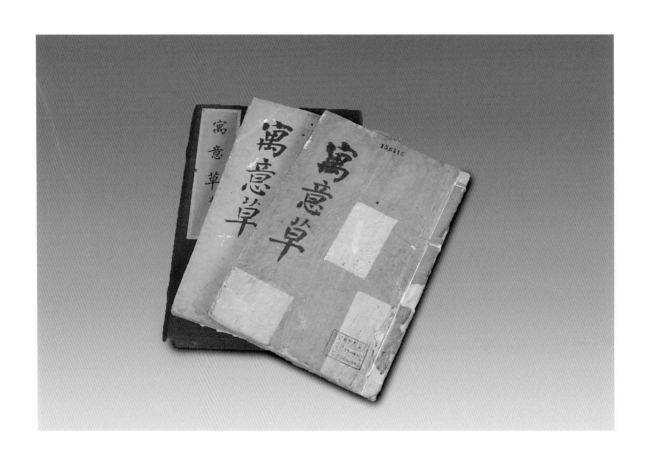

《寓意草》

清

23 厘米 ×15.2 厘米

Yu Yi Cao

Qing Dynasty

23 cm×15.2 cm

线装书，医籍。《寓意草》为清医家喻昌著。为喻昌临证验案笔录，共载六十余复杂病例。该藏本为清光绪年海阳金忠诠手抄本，分上下两册，线装善本。保存基本完整，纸张泛黄，局部磨损有蛀孔。1959 年入藏。

中华医学会 / 上海中医药大学医史博物馆藏

The books were assembled by traditional thread binding method. *Yu Yi Cao* was written by a famous doctor Yu Chang in the Qing Dynasty. The content of the book was the record of about sixty clinical cases of Yu Chang. The books shown in the picture were the hand-written edition by Jin Zongquan during the reign of Emperor Guangxu in the Qing Dynasty. There are two volumes. The books are well preserved with yellowing paper and partial abrasion. The books were collected in 1959.

Preserved in Chinese Medical Association/ Museum of Chinese Medicine, Shanghai University of Traditional Chinese Medicine

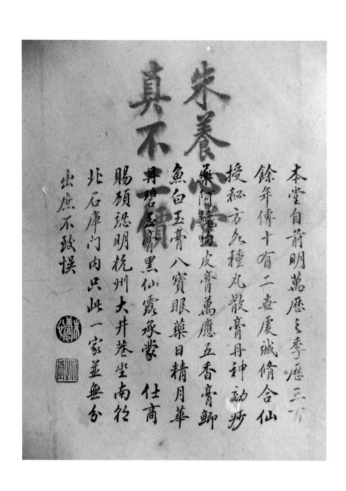

朱养心堂包装纸

清

长 50 厘米，宽 44 厘米

Wrapping Paper of Zhu Yangxin Drugstore

Qing Dynasty

Heigh 50 cm/ Width 44 cm

明代万历年间，伤外科医家朱养心，从浙江余姚迁居杭州，在杭州大井巷口开设朱养心丹膏店。今遗址尚存。

朱德明藏

During the reign of Emperor Wanli of the Qing Dynasty (1573-1620), Zhu Yangxin, a surgeon, moved from Yuyao to Hangzhou, Zhejiang Province, and opened a drugstore named after himself in the Big Well Lane of Hangzhou. The site still remains there today.

Preserved by Zhu Deming

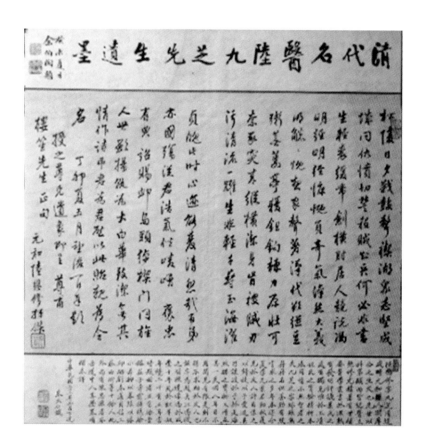

吴尚先行书扇页

清

长 20 厘米，宽 11.5 厘米

Wu Shangxian's Running Script on Fan

Qing Dynasty

Length 20 cm/ Width 11.5 cm

吴尚先，名安业，字师机，晚年署杖潜玉居士，生于清嘉庆十一年九月，殁于光绪十二年八月初六，初本业儒，后侨寓扬州，工书法，擅医学，力主外治法，将其心得著述成书，名为《理瀹骈文》。其除常用膏药外贴外，尚有薰、浸、洗、擦、针灸、按摩等治疗方法。

广东中医药博物馆藏

Wu Shangxian (first name Anye, style name Shiji, pseudonym Zhangqianyu Jushi) was born in September, the 11th year of Emperor Jiaqing's Period in the Qing Dynasty and died on 6 August, the 12th year of Emperor Guangxu's Period. He was good at calligraphy and medicine, especially external treatment. He wrote his ideas into a book named "*Li Lun Pian Wen*" (Theory Prose). In addition to the conventional plaster, there are other treatments like smoke, dip, wash, wipe, acupuncture, and massage.

Preserved in Guangdong Chinese Medicine Museum

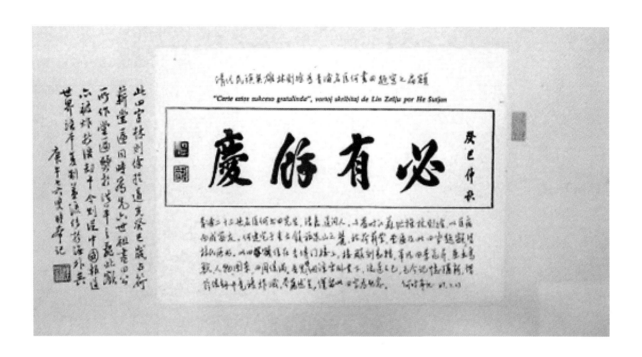

林则徐"必有余庆"匾额

清

镜片：长 61.5 厘米，宽 32.9 厘米

Horizontal Inscribed Board of *Bi You Yu Qing* Written by Lin Zexu

Qing Dynasty

Mounted Piece: Length 61.5 cm/ Width 32.9 cm

镜片，为艺术品，是清代民族英雄林则徐为青浦名医何书田题写的"必有余庆"匾额。何书田，清嘉庆道光年间人，青浦何氏二十三世名医，与当时江苏巡抚林则徐以医病而成密友。何建宅于古重镇福泉山之麓，称荷薪堂，林氏为之题写匾额。镜片左侧、下方有何时希题记。匾额为复印件，已装裱成镜片，保存基本完好。1991年入藏。

中华医学会 / 上海中医药大学医史博物馆藏

It is a horizontal inscribed board of characters "Bi You Yu Qing" written by Lin Zexu, a national hero in the Qing Dynasty, for He Shutian, a famous doctor in Qingpu. He Shutian was the 23th generation doctor of Family. He in Qingpu County. Lin Zexu, the grand coordinator in Jiangsu Province at that time, was his patient before they became good friends. He built his house at the foot of Fuquan Mountain in Guchong County. His house was called He Xin Tang, which received Lin Zexu's handwritten board. He Shixi's inscription was on the left and lowers parts of the piece. This is a copy of the original and has been mounted. It was collected in 1991 and is still in good condition.

Preserved in Chinese Medical Association/ Museum of Chinese Medicine, Shanghai University of Traditional Chinese Medicine

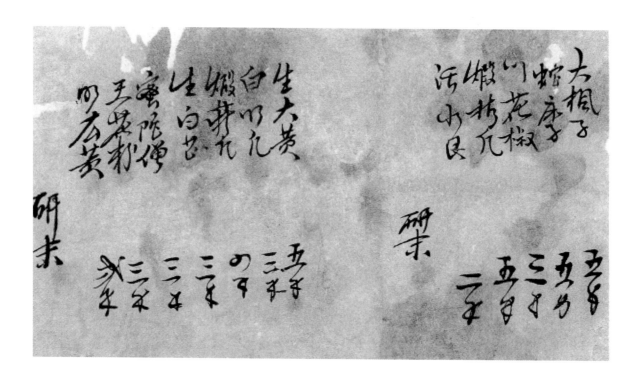

太平天国药方

清

长 20.5 厘米，宽 11.7 厘米

Prescriptions in the Taiping Heavenly Kingdom

Qing Dynasty

Length 20.5 cm/ Width 11.7 cm

图为太平天国高级官员俄天义吴习玖阁内中药处方笺。1996 年 7 月，苏州市红旗区葑门内吴衙场 42 号商业学校出土。

苏州博物馆藏

These are the Chinese medicine prescriptions in the family of Wu Xijiu, a senior official of Taiping Heavenly Kingdom . They were unearthed at a business school (No. 42, Wuyachang, Fengmen) of Hongqi District, Suzhou City, Jiangsu Province.

Preserved in Suzhou Museum

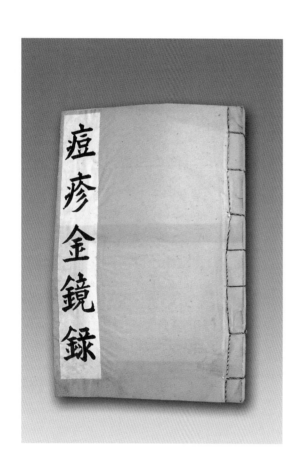

《痘疹金镜录》

清

45 厘米 ×29.8 厘米

Dou Zhen Jin Jing Lu

Qing Dynasty

45 cm×29.8 cm

线装书，医籍，全称《增补痘疹金镜录》，明儿科医学家信州翁仲仁（嘉德）辑著。该藏有清康熙二十九年（庚午年）钱塘仇沄（天一）考证抄录时所作序，为线装精抄本，应为道光年间抄录重刊，抄录人待考。保存基本完整，纸张泛黄，局部磨损有蛀孔。1959 年入藏。

中华医学会 / 上海中医药大学医史博物馆藏

The book *Dou Zhen Jin Jing Lu* (Collected Edition of Exanthema Variolosum) is a thread-bound medical book. The full name of the book is *Zeng Bu Dou Zhen Jin Jing Lu*. The author was Weng Zhongren (Jiade) from Xinzhou County in the Ming Dynasty. This collection included the preface made by Qiu Yun (Tianyi) from Qiantang County when he copied the original edition in the 29th year of the reign of Emperor Kangxi. This thread-bound hardback was probably re-copied in the reign of Emperor Daoguang, and the person who copied it remains to be proven. This collection was almost complete with yellow discolouration. Some parts of it were abrasions with borer holes. It was collected in 1959.

Preserved in Chinese Medical Association/ Museum of Chinese Medicine, Shanghai University of Traditional Chinese Medicine

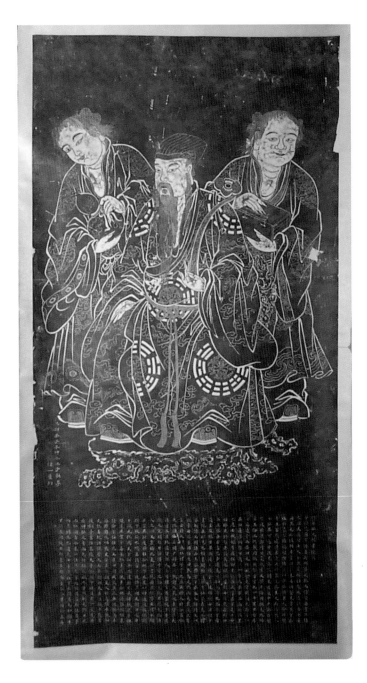

华元化画像碑拓

近现代

卷轴：长 204.2 厘米，宽 83.8 厘米

画芯：长 151.7 厘米，宽 76.1 厘米

Stele Rubbing of Hua Yuanhua's Portrait

Modern Times

Scroll: Length 204.2 cm/ Width 83.8 cm

Painting: Length 151.7 cm/ Width 76.1 cm

卷轴，是拓片。该碑为清道光七年吴郡王仲芬沐
手敬摹、谭一夔刻华元化画像，下有顾千里撰"刻
华仙元化画像记"。该碑由长洲钱安均书，为吴
郡黄华钰仝男国珍所立。此碑藏苏州白莲桥斗姆
阁。拓片已裱成卷轴，纸张泛黄，画面有污迹。
1958 年入藏。

中华医学会 / 上海中医药大学医史博物馆藏

The stele was facsimiled by Wang Zhongfen (born
in Wu County) in the seventh year of Emperor
Daoguang's Period, and carved by Tan Yikui, with
Gu Qianli's essay "Ke Hua Xian Yuan Hua Hua
Xiang Ji" (Record of Engraving Hua Yuanhua's
Portrait). The inscription was hand-written by Qian
Anjun (born in Changzhou County). The stele was
set by Huang Huayu, etc. and preserved in Dou
Mu Pavilion, Bai Lian Bridge in Suzhou City. This
scroll of rubbing has some yellow discolouration
and stains on the paper. It was collected in 1958.
Preserved in Chinese Medical Association/ Museum
of Chinese Medicine, Shanghai University of
Traditional Chinese Medicine

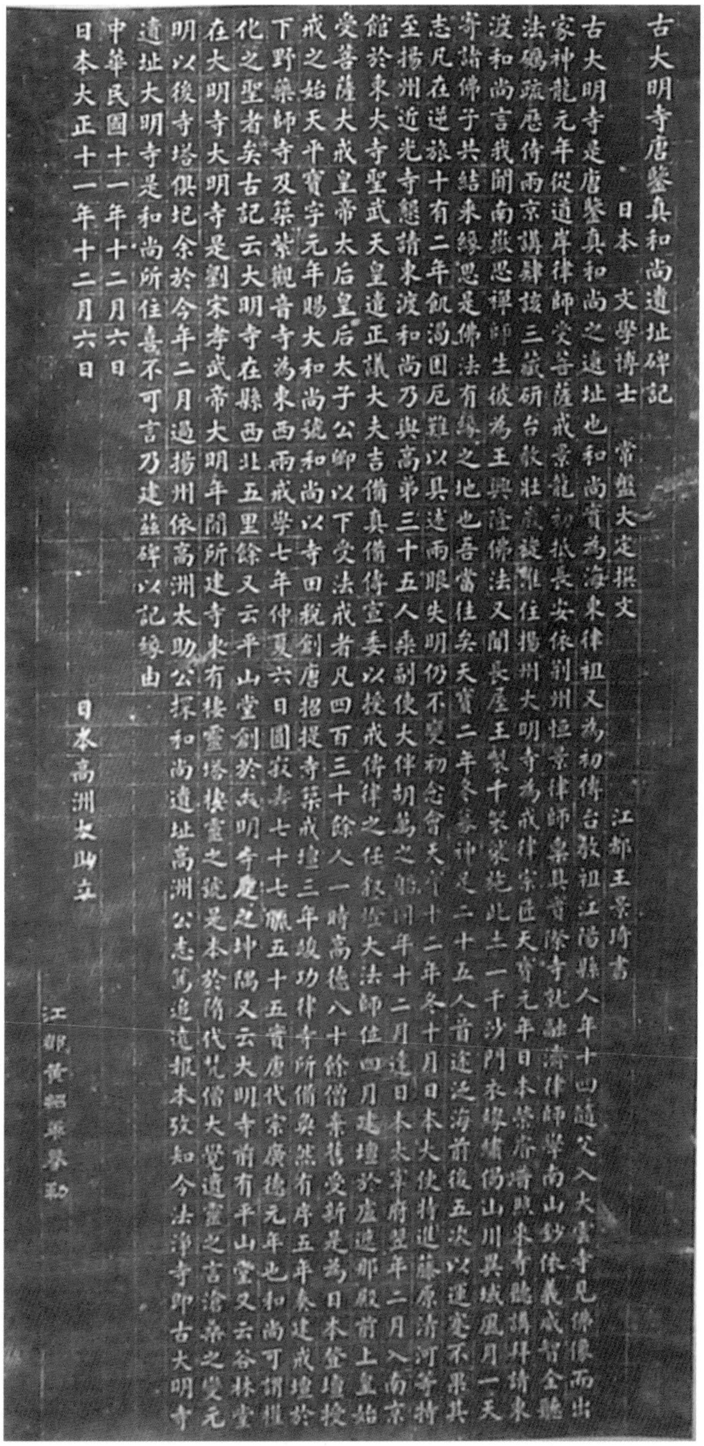

古大明寺唐鉴真和尚遗址碑记拓片

近现代

卷轴：长 211.4 厘米，宽 72.6 厘米

画芯：长 129.1 厘米，宽 60.8 厘米

Stele Rubbing about Monk Jian Zhen in Daming Temple

Modern Times

Scroll: Length 211.4 cm/ Width 72.6 cm

Painting: Length 129.1 cm/ Width 60.8 cm

卷轴，为拓片。该碑记由日本文学博士常盘大定撰文，江都王景琦书，民国十一年十二月六日日本高州太助立，江都黄绍华摹勒。碑文记述古大明寺唐鉴真和尚遗址、鉴真生平事迹和建碑缘由。鉴真（688—763），唐高僧，广陵江阳人，本姓淳于。唐天宝年间东渡日本，传律讲经，传授中医药知识，对日本汉方医药发展有一定影响。拓片已裱成卷轴，纸张泛黄，画面有污迹。1958 年入藏。

中华医学会 / 上海中医药大学医史博物馆藏

This inscription was drafted by Tokiwa Daijyou, a Japanese Doctor in Literature, and written by Wang Jingqi. On 6th December, 11th year of the Republic of China, the stele was erected by Takasu Taisuke from Japan, and carved by Huang Shaohua from Jiangdu. The inscription describes the relics of Monk Jian Zhen in the ancient Daming Temple of the Tang Dynasty, his life story and the reason for the stele erection. Jian Zhen (688–763, surname Chunyu), an eminent monk of the Tang Dynasty, was from Jiangyang, Guangling County. During the Emperor Tianbao's Period of the Tang Dynasty, he went to Japan to preach Buddhism and teach Chinese medical knowledge, which had an impact on the development of the Chinese medicine in Japan. This scroll of rubbing has some yellow discolouration and stains on the paper. It was collected in 1958.

Preserved in Chinese Medical Association/ Museum of Chinese Medicine, Shanghai University of Traditional Chinese Medicine

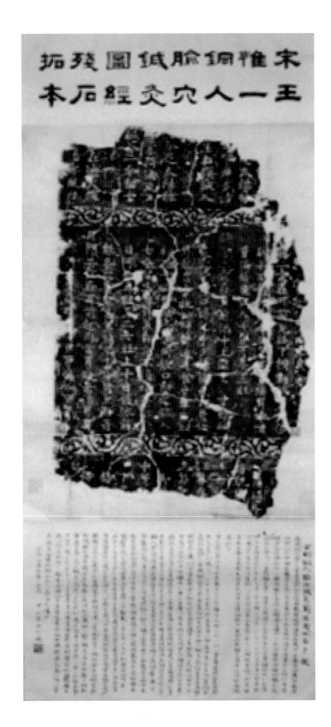

宋代王惟一铜人腧穴针灸图经残石
拓本

近现代

109 厘米×46 厘米

Rubbing of Residual Stone
Inscription of Wang Weiyi's
Acupoints Works

Modern Times

109 cm×46 cm

宋代王惟一著《铜人腧穴针灸图经》，天圣八年，宋政府组织
人员将全书雕成四块石刻，并以石刻为壁建成"针灸石壁堂"
至明代，北宋石刻年久残坏，明太医院镂刻行《铜人经》并刻石，
自此宋代石刻渐沦落，1965—1971 年北京拆除明代北京城墙
时陆续发现三块北宋石刻残石，此即其中一块之拓片。

广东中医药博物馆藏

The author of *Tong Ren Shu Xue Zhen Jiu Tu Jing* (Bronze
Acupoints Acupuncture Figure) is Wang Weiyi in the Song
Dynasty. In the eighth year of Emperor Tiansheng's Period, the
Song government had the book carved in four stone inscriptions
and built "Acupuncture Stone Wall Hall" using these stones as
walls, which remained till the Ming Dynasty. In the Northern Song
Dynasty, the stone inscriptions were in poor condition, therefore,
the imperial hospital of the Ming Dynasty carved "*Tong Ren
Jing*" (Bronze Acupuncture Figure) on stone. From then on, the
stone inscriptions in the Song Dynasty were gradually missing.
In 1965–1971, when Beijing city walls of the Ming Dynasty were
demolished, three residual stone inscriptions in the Northern Song
Dynasty were found, and this is one of them.

Preserved in Guangdong Chinese Medicine Museum

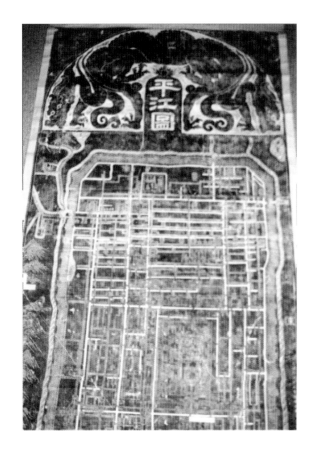

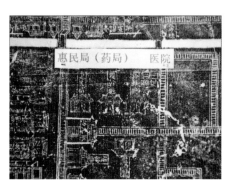

宋代平江图拓片

近现代

整体：长 215 厘米，138 厘米

局部：长 10 厘米，宽 7 厘米

Rubbing of Pingjiang Map in Song Dynasty (Full Figure)

Modern Times

Holistic: Length 215 cm/ Width 138 cm

Part: Length 10 cm/ Width 7 cm

此为宋代平江府（今苏州）地形图，宋理宗绍定二年制，图中有
惠民局医院设置。惠民局是宋代官办的卖药机构。据考证惠民局
医院创建于宋嘉定年间，后来变成了专治囚犯生的"安养"院。
下方局部图为宋代平江府（今苏州）地形图中惠民局医院设置。
1229 年刻成的我国现存最早的城市平面图《平江图》上，可以
看到"医院""惠民局"镌刻于上，这是我国最早出现"医院"
两字的实证资料。

广东中医药博物馆藏

This is a topographic map of Pingjiang Fu (now Suzhou City) in the
Song Dynasty, and was made in the second year of Shaoding Period
under the reign of Emperor Lizong of the Song Dynasty. Medical
Institute of Benevolence was also recorded in the map. Medical
Institute of Benevolence was the official medicine agency in the
Song Dynasty. According to research, the Affiliated Hospital of
Medical Institute of Benevolence was established during the years
of Jiading Period, and afterwards it was transformed into a "nursing
home" for sick prisoners. This is the layout of the Affiliated Hospital
of Medical Institute of Benevolence in topographic map of Pingjiang
Fu (now Suzhou City) in the Song Dynasty. Pingjiang Map, carved
in 1229, is China's earliest existing city plan. In the rubbing it can be
seen the Chinese characters "Yi Yuan" which means "Hospital" and
"Hui Min Ju" which means "Medical Institute of Benevolence". It is
China's earliest material where the term "Yi Yuan" appears.
Preserved in Guangdong Chinese Medicine Museum

明"倪砚香诊"牙章拓片

近现代

印面：长2.8厘米，宽2.8厘米

Rubbing of Tooth Seal "Ni Yan Xiang Zhen"

Modern Times

The Seal Face: Length 2.8cm/ Width2.8cm

方形，为拓片。此印拓阴文篆刻"倪砚香诊"四字，字体工整；原为明代牙章，有兽钮，兽似狮似虎，瞠目露齿，作匍匐状。倪砚香详情待考。拓片基本完好，已装裱成卡片。1958 年入藏。

中华医学会 / 上海中医药大学医史博物馆藏

This rubbing is square. This seal is engraved with neat intaglio "Ni Yan Xiang Zhen". It was a tooth seal in the Ming Dynasty with a knob of beast, which was like a lion and a tiger in a prostrate form with frightening grin. Details about "Ni Yan Xiang" are to be explored. The rubbing is intact and has been mounted into a card. It was collected in 1958.

Preserved in Chinese Medical Association/ Museum of Chinese Medicine, Shanghai University of Traditional Chinese Medicine

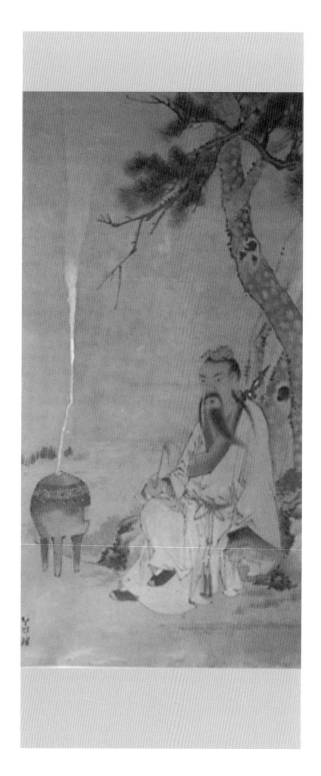

吕纯阳炼丹图

近现代

卷轴：长 159 厘米，宽 65.8 厘米

画芯：长 104.5 厘米，宽 61.8 厘米

Painting of Lü Chunyang and Alchemy

Modern Times

Scroll: Length 159 cm/ Width 65.8 cm

Painting: Length 104.5 cm/ Width 61.8 cm

卷轴为书画。甲申僧所画。画面为吕纯阳手
持甩子安坐在炼丹炉旁炼丹的场面。画已裱
成卷轴，纸张泛黄，画面污迹，上端已撕开。
1957 年入藏。

中华医学会 / 上海中医药大学医史博物馆藏

The picture was painted by Jia Shenseng. In
the picture, Lü Chunyang (a famous Taoist) is
sitting near an alchemy stove with a horsetail
whisk. The rubbing has been made into a
scroll. The scroll of rubbing has some yellow
discoloration and stains on the paper. The upper
part has been torn. It was collected in 1957.
Preserved in Chinese Medical Association/
Museum of Chinese Medicine, Shanghai
University of Traditional Chinese Medicine

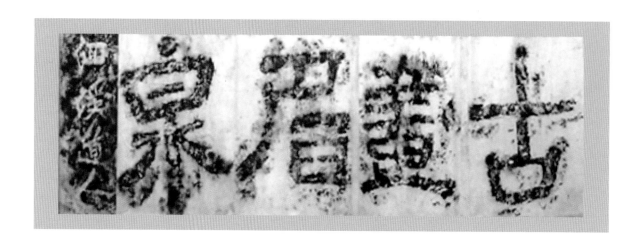

古画眉泉拓本

近现代

卷轴：长 150 厘米，宽 35.5 厘米

画芯：长 103.7 厘米，宽 30 厘米

Rubbing of "Gu Hua Mei Quan"

Modern Times

Scroll: Length 150 cm/ Width 35.5 cm

Rubbing: Length 103.7 cm/ Width 30 cm

卷轴为拓片，为徐灵胎晚年隐居苏州七子山画眉泉所书石刻拓片。拓片已裱成卷轴，纸张泛黄，画面有污迹。1958 年入藏。

中华医学会 / 上海中医药大学医史博物馆藏

It is stonecutting rubbing of characters written by Xu Lingtai in his later life when he lived in seclusion in Huameiquan (Huamei fountain) in Qizi Mountain, Suzhou City. It has been made into a scroll. There are discoloration and stains on the paper. It was collected in 1958.

Preserved in Chinese Medical Association/ Museum of Chinese Medicine, Shanghai University of Traditional Chinese Medicine

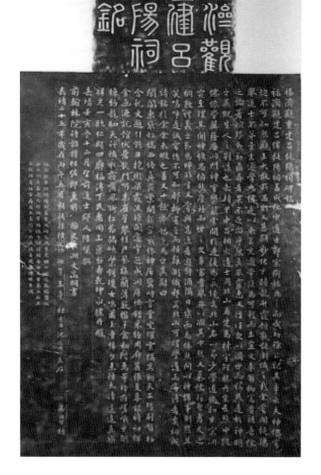

文徵明书重建吕纯阳祠碑拓

近现代

卷轴：长 215.5 厘米，宽 84.5 厘米

画芯：长 150.5 厘米，宽 72 厘米

Rubbing of Stele for Reconstruction of Lü Chunyang Temple

Modern Times

Scroll: Length 215.5 cm/ Width 84.5 cm

Rubbing: Length 150.5 cm/ Width 72 cm

卷轴为拓片。该碑为明嘉靖二十五年文徵明书，行楷体。本藏

是清嘉庆二十四年钱塘陈桂生在福济观吕仙祠重修时临摹重刻

碑之拓片。文徵明（1470—1559），明代江南四大才子之一。

此碑存苏州阊门内福济观。拓片已裱成卷轴，纸张泛黄，画面

有污迹。1958 年入藏。

中华医学会 / 上海中医药大学医史博物馆藏

This inscription was written by Wen Zhengming in regular script
in the 25th year of Jiajing Period in the Ming Dynasty. The picture
shows the rubbing of the inscription facsimiled by Chen Guisheng
(from Qiantang County) in the 24th year of Emperor Jiaqing's
Period in the Qing Dynasty on the reconstruction of Lü Temple
in Fujiguan. Wen Zhengming (1470–1559) was one of the four
greatest talented scholars in the Ming Dynasty in the lower reaches
of the Changjiang River. This stele is preserved in Fujiguan,
Suzhou City. The rubbing has been made into a scroll and there are
yellow discolouration and stains on the paper. It was collected in 1958.
Preserved in Chinese Medical Association/ Museum of Chinese
Medicine, Shanghai University of Traditional Chinese Medicine

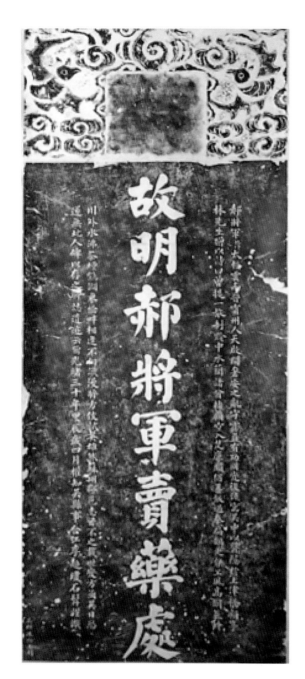

郝将军卖药处碑拓本

近现代

卷轴：长 216.3 厘米，宽 68.2 厘米

画芯：长 145.5 厘米，宽 56 厘米

Rubbing of "Drug Store of General Hao"

Modern Times

Scroll: Length 216.3 cm/ Width 68.2 cm

Rubbing: Length 145.5 cm/ Width 56 cm

卷轴为拓片。该碑记是清光绪三十年（1904）为纪念故明郝将军所立石碑之拓本。碑文楷体"故明郝将军卖药处"两侧有楷体小字注明缘由，左下刻有"吴郡陈伯玉刻"字样。此碑存苏州上津桥。拓片已裱成卷轴，纸张泛黄，画面有污迹。1958年入藏。

中华医学会/上海中医药大学医史博物馆藏

It is a rubbing of stele inscription made in the thirtieth year of Emperor Guangxu's Period in the Qing Dynasty (1904) to commemorate General Hao of the old Ming Dynasty. On both sides of the regular script inscription "Drugs Store of General Hao of the Old Ming Dynasty", there are small-sized regular scripts elaborating the details. On the lower left part were engraved characters meaning "Carved by Chen Boyu from Wu County". The stele is preserved in Shangjin Bridge in Suzhou City. The rubbing has been made into a scroll and there are yellow discolouration and stains on the paper. It was collected in 1958.

Preserved in Chinese Medical Association/ Museum of Chinese Medicine, Shanghai University of Traditional Chinese Medicine

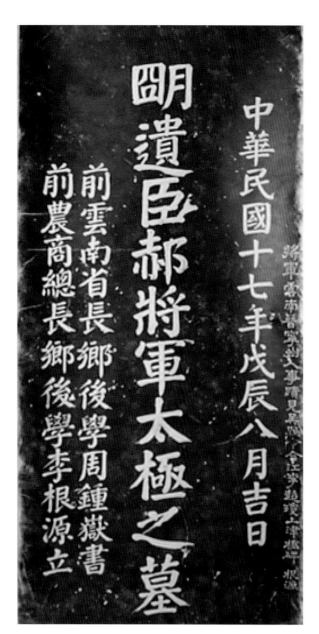

郝将军太极之墓碑拓本

近现代

卷轴：长 207.5 厘米，宽 59.5 厘米

画芯：长 105.3 厘米，宽 46.8 厘米

Rubbing of General Hao's Tombstone

Modern Times

Scroll: Length 207.5 cm/ Width 59.5 cm

Rubbing: Length 105.3 cm/ Width 46.8 cm

卷轴为拓片。该碑是 1928 年，前云南省长乡后学周钟岳书，前农商总长乡后学李根源立。碑文楷体"明遗臣郝将军太极之墓"。其墓位于苏州李继宗巷郝墓。拓片已裱成卷轴，纸张泛黄，画面有污迹。1958 年入藏。

中华医学会／上海中医药大学医史博物馆藏

The stele inscription was written by Zhou Zhongyu, the former governor of Yunnan Province and erected by Li Genyuan, the former official of agriculture and commerce in the 17th year of the Republic of China. The inscription in regular script says "Tomb of General Hao of the Old Ming Dynasty". It is located in Hao tomb, Li Jizong Lane, Suzhou City. The rubbing has been made into a scroll and there are yellow discolouration and stains on the paper. It was collected in 1958.

Preserved in Chinese Medical Association/ Museum of Chinese Medicine, Shanghai University of Traditional Chinese Medicine

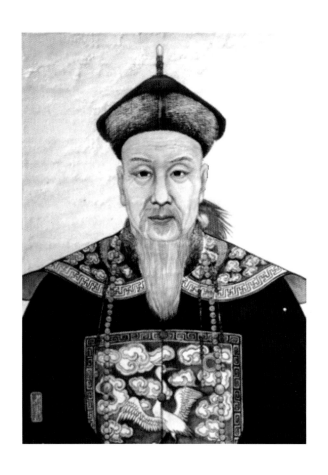

徐灵胎像

近现代

长 39 厘米，宽 27 厘米

Portrait of Xu Lingtai

Modern Times

Length 39 cm/ Width 27 cm

徐大椿，又名大业，字灵胎，晚号加溪老人，清代江苏吴江县人。其自幼习儒，旁及诸子百家，年近三十，因家人多病而致力医学，久之妙悟医理，遂悬壶于世。即使危重病患，亦能药到病除。其平生好著述，今存著有《难经经释》《神农本草经百种录》《医贯砭》《医学源流论》等。

广东中医药博物馆藏

Xu Dachun (also called Daye, styled name Lingtai and Jiaxi Laoren in later life) was from Wujiang County, Jiangsu Province in the Qing Dynasty. He had learned Confucianism and also theories of all classes of scholars since childhood. For nearly 30 years, he was engaged in medical practice for the sake of his family's health. Year after year, he became a master in medicine and then became famous in the world. He could even cure those who were severely sick. Xu also loved to write during his life. His existent works include *Nan Jing Jing Bian* (Nanjing Notes), *Shen Nong Ben Cao Jing Bai Zhong Lu* (Records of Shen Nong's Herbal), *Yi Guan Bian*(Commentaries on Book Yi Guan), and *Yi Xue Yuan Liu Lun* (On Origins of Medicine) .

Preserved in Guangdong Chinese Medicine Museum

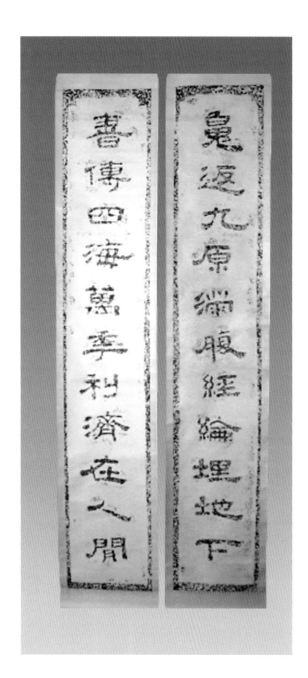

徐灵胎墓门长联拓本

近现代

卷轴：长 218 厘米，宽 35.2 厘米

画芯：长 186.5 厘米，宽 29.8 厘米

Rubbing of Long Couplets on Xu Lingtai's Tomb

Modern Times

Scroll：Length 218 cm/ Width 35.2 cm

Rubbing：Length 186.5 cm/ Width 29.8 cm

卷轴为徐灵胎墓门石刻对联拓片。对联内容为隶书"魄返九原满腹经纶埋地下，书传四海万季利济在人间"。徐大椿（1693—1771），字灵胎，江苏吴江（今苏州）人。清代名医，博览方书，精研医理。乾隆二十六年及三十六年两次应招入宫治病。其平生著述甚丰，主要有《医学源流论》《伤寒类方》《医贯砭》《兰台轨范》《难经注释》等。拓片已裱成卷轴，纸张泛黄，画面有污迹。1958 年入藏。

中华医学会 / 上海中医药大学医史博物馆藏

This stonecutting couplets on Xu Lingtai's tomb arch were written in official script saying that a learned man was buried under the ground, but his works were still on earth which could benefit many people. Xu Dachun (1693–1771, styled name Lingtai) was from Wujiang County (now as Suzhou City), in Jiangsu Province. He was a famous doctor in the Qing Dynasty with good knowledge in prescriptions and medical theory. He was summoned twice to treat people in the imperial palace in the 26th and 36th year of Emperor Qianlong's Period in the Qing Dynasty. Among his abundant medical works, the most well-known are *Yi Xue Yuan Liu Lun* (On Medical Origin), *Shang Han Lei Fang* (Prescriptions on Typhia), *Yi Guan Bian* (Commentaries on Book Yi Guan), *Lan Tai Gui Fan* (*Lantai Criteria*) and *Nan Jing Zhu Shi* (Nanjing Notes). The rubbing has been made into scrolls and there are some yellow discoloration and stains on the paper. It was collected in 1958.

Preserved in Chinese Medical Association/ Museum of Chinese Medicine, Shanghai University of Traditional Chinese Medicine

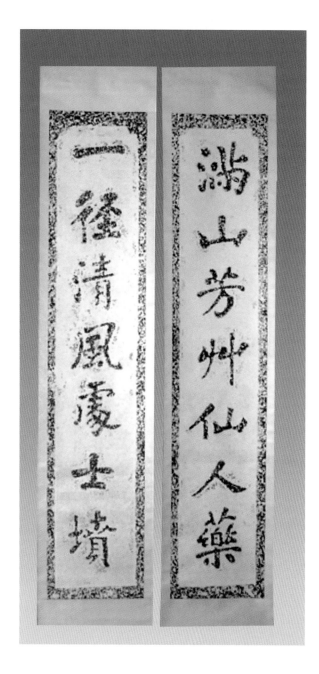

徐灵胎墓门短联拓本

近现代

卷轴：长 178.8 厘米，宽 33.4 厘米

画芯：长 143.2 厘米，宽 27.6 厘米

Rubbing of Short Couplets on Xu Lingtai's Tomb

Modern Times

Scroll：Length 178.8 cm/ Width 33.4 cm

Rubbing: Length 143.2 cm/ Width 27.6 cm

卷轴，为徐灵胎墓门石刻对联拓片。对联内容为
楷书"满山芳草仙人药，一径清风处士坟"。拓
片已裱成卷轴，纸张泛黄，画面有污迹。1958 年
入藏。

中华医学会 / 上海中医药大学医史博物馆藏

The stonecutting couplets on Xu Lingtai's tomb
arch were written in regular script, saying that
there were herbal medicines on the mountain, and
the tomb for this gentleman was in the breeze. The
rubbing has been made into scrolls and there are
some yellow discolouration and stains on the paper.
It was collected in 1958.

Preserved in Chinese Medical Association/ Museum
of Chinese Medicine, Shanghai University of
Traditional Chinese Medicine

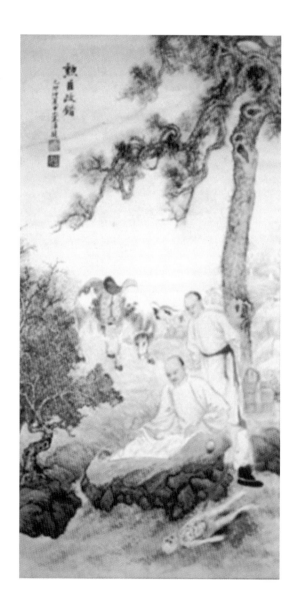

勋臣改错图挂画

近现代

64 厘米 ×32 厘米

A Wall Picture of Xunchen Correcting Medical Errors

Modern Times

64 cm×32 cm

王清任，字勋臣，清代直隶玉田人（今河北玉田人），精医术，名噪京师，注重研究人体脏腑，"业医诊病，当先明脏腑"。而当时医家多注重考证、校注，脏腑之说多因袭前人之说。清任立志重绘人体脏腑图，曾不避污秽，连续十日对义冢中破腹露脏尸体进行细致观察并描绘其形态，前后历经四十年最终绘脏腑全图，写成《医林改错》。

广东中医药博物馆藏

Wang Qingren (courtesy name Xunchen), born in Yutian County of Zhili Province (now Yutian County of Hebei Province) in the Qing Dynasty, was a famous doctor in the capital city. He paid attention to the research on internal organs, advocating that doctors should examine function of patients' organs before diagnosis and treatment. However, at that time, most doctors emphasized on textual research, collation and annotation, and they often referred to the previous theories on organs. Instead, Wang Qingren was determined to draw the picture of human organs again, and had carefully observed corpses with broken belly for ten days in the cemetery without fearing the dirtiness and depicted the forms of organs. After 40 years of effort, he finally finished the pictures of human organs and wrote "Yi Lin Gai Cuo" (*Correction of the Errors of Medical Books*). Preserved in Guangdong Chinese Medicine Museum

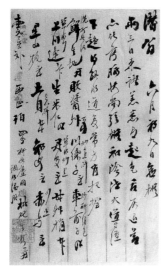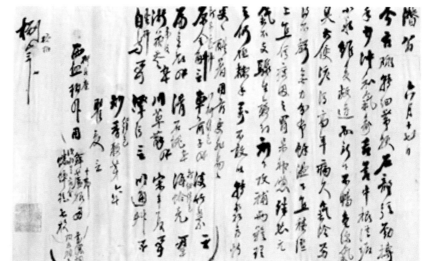

曹沧洲处方

近现代

长 26 厘米，宽 12 厘米

Prescriptions Written by Cao Cangzhou

Modern Times

Length 26 cm/ Width 12 cm

曹沧洲（1849-1931），晚清江苏名医，居
江苏苏州姑苏、间门西街，祖父曹云洲，父
亲曹承洲皆精内科方脉，兼通外科。1907 年
与陈莲舫应召入京为光绪帝治病，其子孙亦
精医。

上海中医药博物馆藏

Cao Cangzhou (1849-1931) was a famous
doctor from Changmen West Street, Gusu
District, Suzhou City of Jiangsu Province.
His grandfather Cao Yunzhou and father Cao
Chengzhou were both proficient in internal
medicine and medical surgery. He came to
the Forbidden City with Chen Lianfang in
1907 to treat the Emperor Guangxu. His
descendants were also proficient in medicine.
Preserved in Shanghai Museum of Traditional
Chinese Medicine

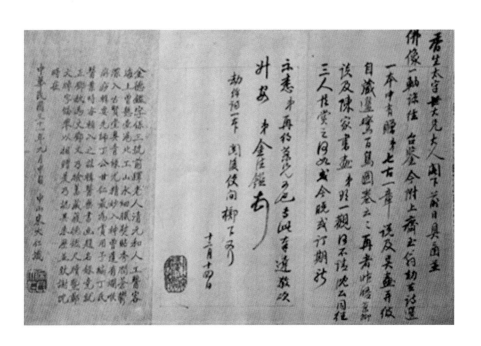

清代医家金德鉴手迹

近现代

14 厘米 ×9 厘米

Handwriting of Jin Dejian

Modern Times

14 cm×9 cm

金德鉴，清代江苏元和县人，精于医学，留心喉科，辑有《焦氏喉科枕秘》二卷、《烂喉丹痧辑要》一卷，今存。

广州中医药博物馆藏

Jin Dejian, born in Yuanhe County of Jiangsu Province, was proficient in medical science and had paid special attention to laryngology. He had written a two-volume book, *Jiao Shi Hou Ke Zhen Mi* (a famous writing of laryngology) and a one-volume book, *Lan Hou Dan Sha Ji Yao* (a medical book of the treatment on an acute infectious disease with the symptom of scarlet fever and swelling throat). These books are preserved until today.

Preserved in Guangdong Chinese Medicine Museum

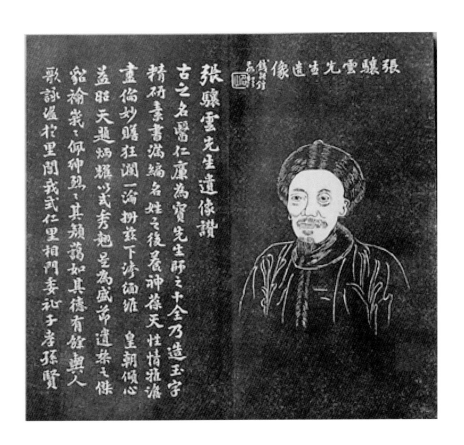

张骧云先生遗像及赞文拓片

近现代

长 29.6 厘米，宽 15.5 厘米

Rubbing of Zhang Xiangyun's Portait and Eulogy

Modern Times

Length 29.6 cm/ Width 15.5 cm

长方形拓片，全称"张骧云像传拓本附家传"，深兰色绸面装帧。该页为第一页，除画像外有嘉兴金蓉镜于丙寅年（1926）题《张骧云先生遗像赞》一文。张骧云（1855－1925），又名世镳，字君相，晚号冰壶，上海人，出生医学世家，以善治伤寒而闻名沪上，有"一帖药"之称，且重医德，中年因患重疾，两耳失聪，人称"张聋（peng）"而声名益盛。其著有《君相诊余随笔》文稿，其子孙中从医者亦常被人尊之为"小聋（peng）"。保存完好。1958 年入藏。

中华医学会 / 上海中医药大学医史博物馆藏

The rubbing, with the full name of "Zhang Xiangyun Xiang Chuan Ta Ben Fu Jia Chuan" (a handed-down rubbing of portrait and biography of Zhang Xiangyun), is bound with dark blue silk cover. This is the first page, on which are the portrait of Zhang Xiangyun and an essay with the title "Zhang Xiangyun Xian Sheng Yi Xiang Zan"(*Culogy of Mr. Zhang Xiangyun*) written by Jin Jingrong (an official in the late Qing Dynasty) from Jiaxing County in the year 1926. Zhang Xiangyun (1855–1925), with alternate name Shilu, courtesy name Junxiang and assumed name Binghu in his old age, was born in a medical family in Shanghai City. He was not only a doctor who was famous for curing exogenous febrile diseases with only one prescription of medicine, but was also well-known for his medical ethics. In his middle age, due to serious disease, he lost his hearing and was then known as "Zhang Peng (meaning deaf)". Zhang Xiangyun has a written manuscript of *Jun Xiang Zhen Yu Sui Bi* (manuscript of Zhang Xiangyun's diagnosis and treatment). His descendants who also became doctors were addressed as "Xiao Peng". This rubbing was collected in the year 1958 and is preserved in good condition.
Preserved in Chinese Medical Association/ Museum of Chinese Medicine, Shanghai University of Traditional Chinese Medicine

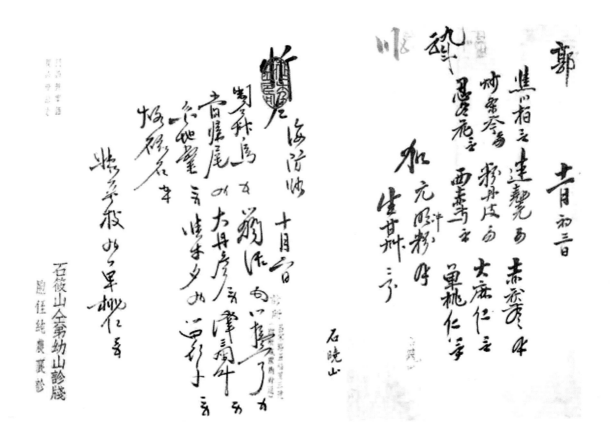

石晓山及其子石筱山处方

近现代

图左为筱山方，长 24 厘米，宽 15 厘米

图右为晓山方，长 23.5 厘米，宽 14.5 厘米

Prescriptions Written by Shi Xiaozhan and His Son

Modern Times

Left Picture: Length 24 cm/ Width 15 cm

Right Picture：Length 23.5 cm/ Width 14.5 cm

石晓山原名石荣宗 (1859—1928), 江苏无锡

人, 伤科名医石兰田之子, 得父传, 兼习针灸、

外科。石筱山为其子, 也精伤骨科。

上海中医药博物馆藏

The right picture is the inscription written by
Shi Xiaoshan, while the left is the inscription
written by his son Jr. Shi Xiaoshan. The father
Shi Xiaoshan (1859-1928, original name
Shi Rongzong, born in Wuxi City, Zhejiang
Province), was the son of Shi Lantian, a famous
traumatologist. Under his father's careful
cultivation, he learnt acupuncture, moxibustion
and surgical skills. The son Shi Xiaoshan Jr.
was also skillful at orthopedics.
Preserved in Shanghai Museum of Traditional
Chinese Medicine

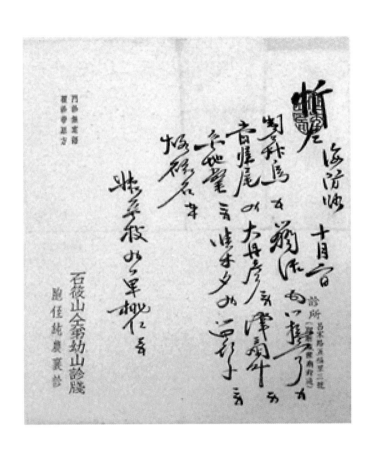

石筱山处方

近现代

处方：长 27.2 厘米，宽 19 厘米

镜片：21.3 厘米 ×32.5 厘米

Prescription Written by Jr Shi Xiaoshan

Modern Times

Prescription: Length 27.2 cm/ Width 19 cm

Mounted piece: Length 32.5 cm/ Width 21.3 cm

该藏是石氏吕宋路五福里三号诊所为忻左医病所开出处方，落款有"石筱山仝弟幼山诊牋"和"胞侄纯农襄诊"。处方充分反映石氏伤科遣方用药特点。石筱山（1904—1964），原名瑞昌，字熙候，无锡人，石氏伤科三世传人。石氏伤科始于道光，其祖父蓝田精武术，能理伤正骨，行医乡里。父晓山，自幼习武，兼理医业。石筱山早年就读于上海神州中医专门学校，后随父学医，继承家传，采各家所长，成为江南伤科一大流派。已装裱成镜片，保存基本完好。1991 年入藏。

中华医学会 / 上海中医药大学医史博物馆藏

This prescription was made for Xin Zuo by No. 3 Clinic of Family Shi in Wufu Alley, Lüsong Street, with signature "Shi Xiaoshan Tong Di You Shan Zhen Jian" (Shi Xiaoshan and his younger brother Youshan made this prescription) and "Bao Zhi Chun Nong Xiang Zhen" (his nephew Chunnong assisted them to diagnose". This prescription completely reflected Shi's features in choosing medicine. Shi Xiaoshan Jr. (1904–1964, original name Ruichang, courtesy name Xihou, born in Wuxi City) was the third-generation heir who passed on medical skills of Shi's department of traumatology. Shi's department of traumatology originated during the reign of Emperor Daoguang. Shi Lantian, the grandfather who was proficient in martial art, possessed the medical skills of bone-setting and curing injuries. Shi Xiaoshan the father, learnt martial art from childhood and practiced medicine at the same time. Shi Xiaoshan Jr. studied in Shanghai Shenzhou Academy of Tradition Chinese Medicine in his early age. Soon afterwards, he learnt medicine with his father, integrated strong points of all classes and established a major school of department of traumatology in regions south of the Yangtze river. This prescription was mounted into a picture frame. It was collected in the year 1991 and is preserved in basically good condition.

Preserved in Chinese Medical Association/ Museum of Chinese Medicine, Shanghai University of Traditional Chinese Medicine

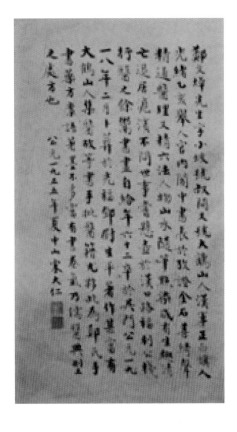
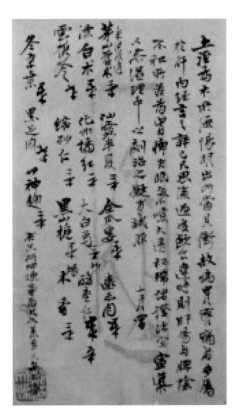

名医赵文焯药方墨迹

近现代

23.5 厘米 ×13 厘米

Handwritten Prescription of Zhao Wenzhuo

Modern Times

23.5 cm×13 cm

长方形。赵文焯，清末民初人，精通医理，

又擅人物山水画，曾官至内阁中书。清亡，

曾悬壶于沪上。此为郑氏手书药方按语。

广东中医药博物馆藏

This rectangular prescription was written by
Zhao Wenzhuo, a famous doctor who lived in
the late Qing Dynasty and the early period of
the Republic of China. He had good knowledge
of medical theory and was proficient in figure
painting and landscape painting. He was once
appointed as Nei Ge Zhong Shu (an official
position in charge of recording and translating
in the Qing Dynasty). After the termination
of the Qing Dynasty, he practiced medicine
in Shanghai. This is the note and comment of
Zheng's handwritten prescriptions.

Preserved in Guangdong Chinese Medicine
Museum

丁福宝石章印蜕

近现代

长 28.5 厘米，宽 18 厘米

Print of Ding Fubao's Stone Seal

Modern Times

Length 28.5 cm/ Width 18 cm

长方形，为印蜕。原章刻"丁福宝读书记"六字，阳文，为上海篆刻名家徐星洲所刻，石料为寿山石。丁福宝（1874—1952），字仲祐，江苏无锡人，对中西医均有研究，编辑《中西医刊》，对西医在中国传播多有贡献。保存基本完好。1961 年入藏。

中华医学会 / 上海中医药大学医史博物馆藏

The shape of this print is rectangular. The original Shoushan-stone seal, made by Xu Xingzhou (a famous engraver in Shanghai), is carved with six protruded characters of "Ding Fu Bao Du Shu Ji". Ding Fubao (1874–1952), with courtesy name of Zhongyou and born in Wuxi of Jiangsu Province, was a medical scholar who has made research on both traditional Chinese medicine and western medicine. He edited "Zhong Xi Yi Kan"(*journal of traditional Chinese and western medicine*) and made great contribution to the popularization of western medicine in China. This print was collected in 1961. It is kept in basically good condition.

Preserved in Chinese Medical Association/ Museum of Chinese Medicine, Shanghai University of Traditional Chinese Medicine

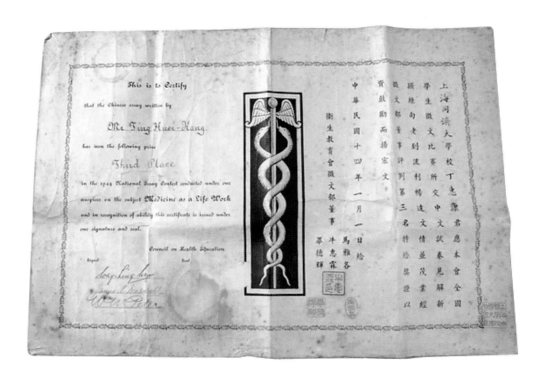

丁惠康征文获奖证书

近现代

46 厘米 ×30.8 厘米

Ding Huikang's Honor Certificate in Essay Competition

Modern Times

46 cm×30.8 cm

长方形，为奖励证书，是 1925 年 1 月 1 日卫生教育会征文部颁发给上海同济大学丁惠康征文获第三名的奖励证书。该证书中英文对照，中部有医标图案，另有征文部董事牛惠霖等落款和签章。保存基本完好。1958 年入藏。

中华医学会 / 上海中医药大学医史博物馆藏

This rectangular honor certificate, made by the essay-soliciting department of Ministry of Health and Education on January 1st in the 14th year of the Republic of China, was awarded to Ding Huikang from Shanghai Tongji University for the 3rd prize in essay competition. This certificate was written in both Chinese and English with a medical symbol in the middle as well as the signatures and seals of the department director, Niu Huilin and others. This certificate was collected in the year 1958. It is kept in basically good condition. Preserved in Chinese Medical Association/ Museum of Chinese Medicine, Shanghai University of Traditional Chinese Medicine

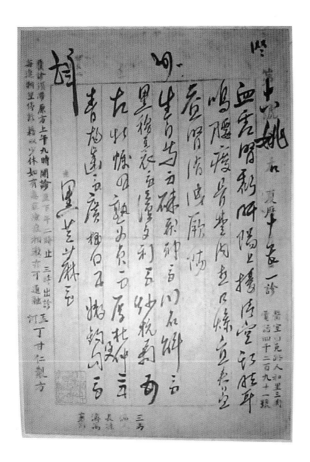

丁甘仁处方

近现代

长 26 厘米，宽 18 厘米

Prescription Written by Ding Ganren

Modern Times

Length 26 cm/ Width 18 cm

长方形，为处方，用丁甘仁专用处方笺写成，是丁甘仁先生为"姚右"所开处方，左下印有"丁甘仁制方"字样。保存完好。1959 年入藏。

中华医学会 / 上海中医药大学医史博物馆藏

This rectangular prescription was written by Ding Ganren on his special prescription-paper for patient Yao You. On the left bottom, there were print characters of "Ding Ganren Zhi Fang" (prescription written by Ding Ganren). This prescription was collected in 1959 and is preserved in good condition.

Preserved in Chinese Medical Association/ Museum of Chinese Medicine, Shanghai University of Traditional Chinese Medicine

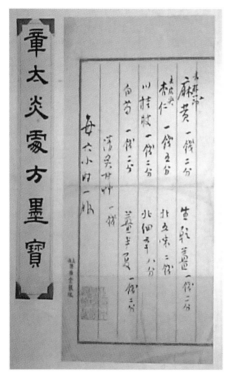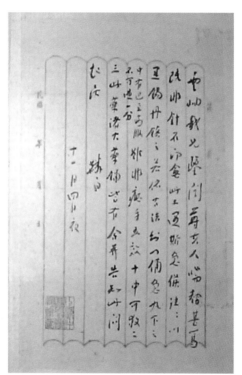

章太炎脉案及处方

近现代

25.5 厘米 ×13 厘米

Diagnosis and Prescription Written by Zhang Taiyan

Modern Times

25.5 cm×13 cm

长方形，为处方，是章氏为余云岫夫人诊疾
的脉案和处方。保存完好。1955 年入藏。

中华医学会 / 上海中医药大学医史博物馆藏

The rectangular diagnosis and prescription were
made by Zhang Tai Yan for Yu Yunxiu's wife.
They were collected in 1955 and are kept in
good condition.

Preserved in Chinese Medical Association/
Museum of Chinese Medicine, Shanghai
University of Traditional Chinese Medicine

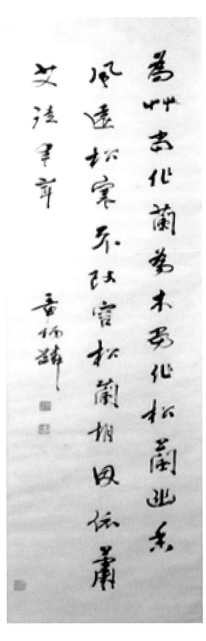

章太炎行草立轴

近现代

卷轴：长 241.3 厘米，宽 60.1 厘米

画芯：长 145.5 厘米，宽 39.9 厘米

Vertical Scroll of Calligraphy by Zhang Taiyan

Modern Times

Scroll: Length 241.3 cm/ Width 60.1 cm

Calligraphy: Length 145.5 cm / Width 39.9 cm

卷轴，艺术品，为章太炎所书行草松蘭诗，左下有"张炳麟"及"太炎"钤记。章太炎（1869—1936），名炳麟，字枚叔，浙江余杭人，近代民主革命家，思想家。博览群书，精诸子百家，对中医理论有独特见解，反对废止中医，也反对中医完全守旧，撰有医著《章太炎医论》（1938）。已裱成卷轴，纸张泛黄，画面有污迹。1959 年入藏。

中华医学会 / 上海中医药大学医史博物馆藏

This is a poem of pine and orchid written in running and grass style by Zhang Taiyan. On the left bottom of the scroll, there are seals of "Zhang Binglin" and "Taiyan". Zhang Taiyan (1869–1936, given name Binglin, courtesy name Meishu) was born in Yuhang County, Jiangsu Province. He was a democratic revolutionist and thinker in the modern times who was well-versed in books, and had a good knowledge of various schools of thoughts. Holding a unique perspective of traditional Chinese medicine, Zhang Taiyan proposed neither its abolishment nor the complete adherence to its past practices. In the year 1938, he wrote famous medical work *Zhang Taiyan Yi Lun*. This handwriting of poem is mounted into scroll while its paper has yellow discolouration and stains on it. This scroll was collected in 1959.

Preserved in Chinese Medical Association/ Museum of Chinese Medicine, Shanghai University of Traditional Chinese Medicine

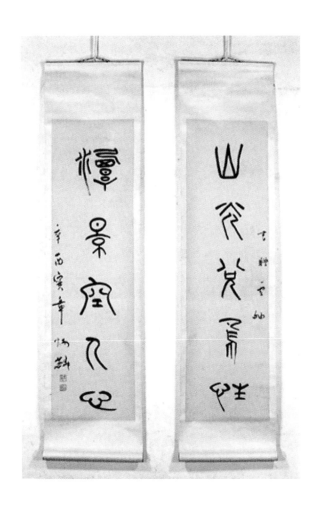

章太炎篆书五言联

近现代

长 13 厘米，宽 2.5 厘米

系章太炎书赠余云岫的对联。联句为："山光兑鸟性，潭景空人心。"

上海中医药博物馆藏

Seal-script Couplets by Zhang Taiyan

Modern Times

Length 13 cm/ Width 2.5 cm

This pair of couplets, written by Zhang Taiyan (a democratic revolutionist, thinker and outstanding scholar), was a gift for Yu Yunxiu (a famous Chinese doctor). Sentences of "Shan Guang Yue Niao Xing, Tan Jing Kong Ren Xin" (a scenery description) were written on the couplets.

Preserved in Shanghai Museum of Traditional Chinese Medicine

夏应堂医案

近现代

长 26 厘米，宽 17.5 厘米

此为夏应堂医治宝源里病人邱氏偏对口医案一则。

上海中医药博物馆藏

Medical Record Written by Xia Yingtang

Modern Times

Length 26 cm/ Width 17.5 cm

This is a medical record written by Xia Yingtang when he treated a patient named Qiu from Bao Yuanli for off-center brain flat-abscess.

Preserved in Shanghai Museum of Traditional Chinese Medicine

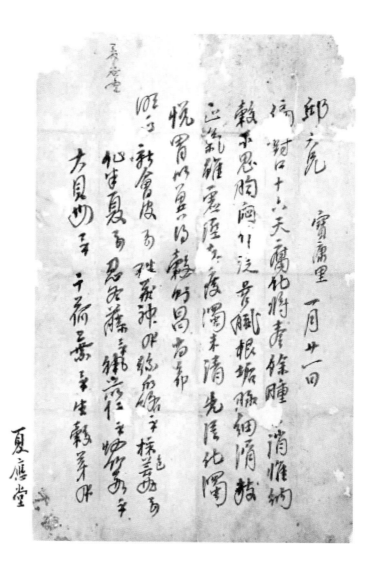

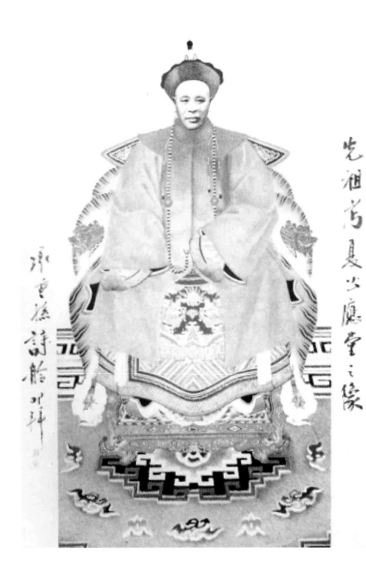

夏应堂画像

近现代

长 160 厘米，宽 66 厘米

Portrait of Xia Yingtang

Modern Times

Length 160 cm/ Width 66 cm

夏应堂（1871—1936），名绍廷，江苏江都县人。居上海，以医问世，与丁甘仁等创办上海中医专门学校。1908 年应"同盟会"之邀赴日本，筹划上海革命运动。夏诗吟捐赠。

上海中医药博物馆藏

Xia Yingtang (1871–1936, given name Shaoting) was born in Jiangdu County, Jiangsu Province. He lived in Shanghai and was well-known as a doctor. He founded the Shanghai Traditional Chinese Medicine Specialized School with Ding Ganren and others, and went to Japan to plan for Shanghai revolutionary movement at the invitation of "Chinese Revolutionary League". The portrait was donated by Xia Shiyin.

Preserved in Shanghai Museum of Traditional Chinese Medicine

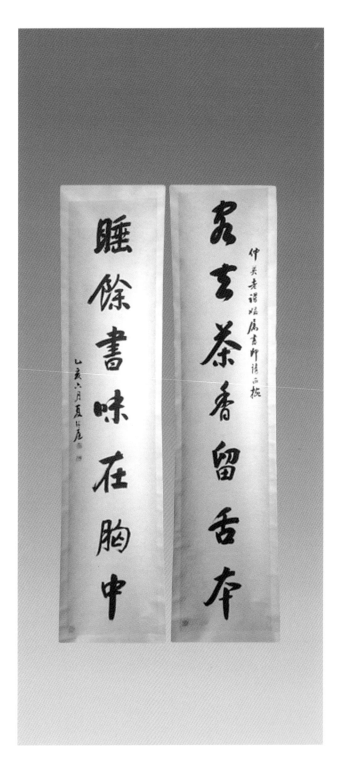

夏应堂书对联

近现代

卷轴：长 200.5 厘米，宽 42.1 厘米

画芯：长 165.5 厘米，宽 34.8 厘米

Couplets Written by Xia Yingtang

Modern Times

Scroll: Length 200.5 cm/ Width 42.1 cm

Couplet: Length 165.5 cm/ Width 34.8 cm

卷轴，为书画，是夏应堂所书行楷对联。对联内容为"尽去茶香留舌本，睡余书味在胸中"，乙亥（1935）年六月书。落有"夏绍庭"印记。夏应堂，江苏江都人，自幼习医，行医45年，经验丰富，疗效卓著，临证用药以轻灵见长，处方精要平稳，看似寻常，恰到好处。门人所著《九芝山馆集方》可窥其医术端倪。已裱成卷轴，纸张泛黄，画面有污迹。1960年入藏。

中华医学会 / 上海中医药大学医史博物馆藏

This is a couplet in running script written by Xia Yingtang. The couplet transcribes a poetic sentence, which means after drinking tea with guests, the tea aroma still remains on your tongue, and when you wake up after reading books, the booky atmosphere still remains in your heart. This couplet was written in June 1935, with a seal "Xia Shaoting". Xia Yingtang was born in Jiangdu City, Jiangsu Province. He had been studying Traditional Chinese Medicine since childhood, and had been practicing medicine for 45 years; therefore, he was very experienced in the treatment of disease. His prescription and medication are common but proper. From the book of *Jiu Zhi Shan Guan Ji Fang* (a medical book on internal medicine) written by his followers, we can know his academic ideas. This prescription has been mounted into a scroll, and there are some stains on the yellowed paper. It was collected in 1960.

Preserved in Chinese Medical Association/Museum of Chinese Medicine, Shanghai University of Traditional Chinese Medicine

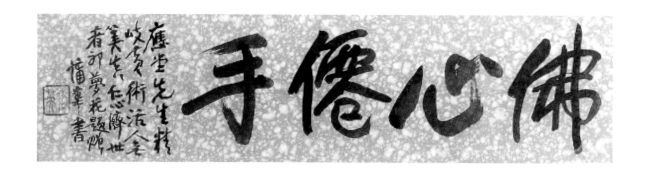

蒲华题"佛心仙手"横额

近现代

长 121 厘米，宽 31.3 厘米

蒲华，海上画派代表人物之一，精书、画。此系他为夏应堂所书。

上海中医药博物馆藏

Banner with characters "Fuo Xin Xian Shou" by Pu Hua

Modern Times

Length 121 cm/ Width 31.3 cm

Pu Hua is one of the representatives of the Shanghai school artists. He was proficient in painting and calligraphy. This is the calligraphy he wrote for Xia Yingtang.

Preserved in Shanghai Museum of Traditional Chinese Medicine

陈筱宝处方

近现代

26.8 厘米 ×21 厘米

长方形，为处方。已装裱成册页，处方多处涂抹，未见患者名及款识，疑为处方之一部分。表面折痕严重。1965 年入藏。

中华医学会 / 上海中医药大学医史博物馆藏

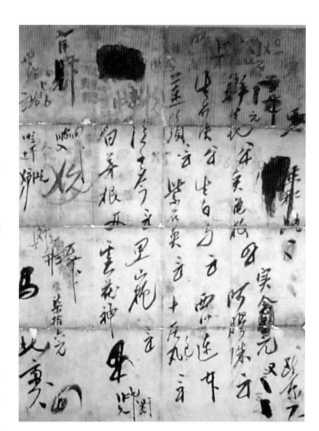

Prescription Written by Chen Xiaobao

Modern Times

26.8 cm×21 cm

This rectangular prescription has been mounted into an album. There were many corrections on the prescription without patient's name and inscriptions, so it seems like one part of the whole prescription. The surface has deep creases. It was collected in 1965.

Preserved in Chinese Medical Association/Museum of Chinese Medicine, Shanghai University of Traditional Chinese Medicine

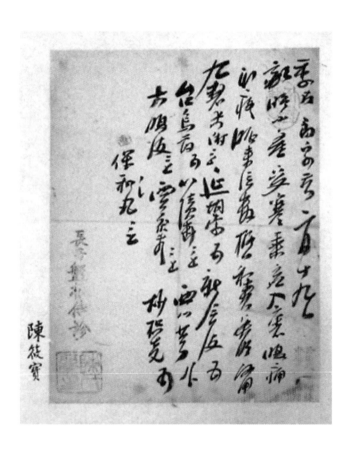

陈筱宝处方

近现代

处方：长 24.3 厘米 ，宽 17.2 厘米

镜片：32.5 厘米 ×21.3 厘米

Prescription Written by Chen Xiaobao

Modern Times

Prescription: Length 24.3 cm/ Width 17.2 cm

Frame: 32.5 cm×21.3 cm

镜片，为处方。该处方上有"长子盘根侍诊"字样，盖"陈氏丽生"朱文印。陈筱宝（1873—1937），名云龙，号丽生，浙江海盐人，幼受父传，习医于妇科名家诸香泉。中年得宋代医家陈素庵《妇科医要》，潜心研读，医道大进。行医40年，临证经验丰富，对妇科有独见，是近现代著名中医妇科医家。已装裱成镜片，保存基本完好。1991年入藏。

中华医学会／上海中医药大学医史博物馆藏

This prescription was mounted in frame. It is inscribed with characters "Chang Zi Pan Gen Shi Zhen" and signed with a seal "Chen Shi Li Sheng". Chen Xiaobao (1873–1937, courtesy name Yun Long, pseudonym name Li Sheng) was born in Haiyan County, Zhejiang Province. He had been studying Traditional Chinese Medicine since childhood and studied from the famous gynecologist Zhu Xiangquan. In middle age, after he studied the book *Fu Ke Yi Yao* (a medical book on gynecology) written by doctor Chen Su'an of the Song Dynasty, his knowledge was improved quickly. He had been practicing medicine for 45 years; therefore, he had rich clinical experience and extraordinary ideas on gynecology. Chen Xiaobao is a well-known gynecologist in modern times. This prescription has been framed. It was collected in 1991 and is preserved well.
Preserved in Chinese Medical Association/Museum of Chinese Medicine, Shanghai University of Traditional Chinese Medicine

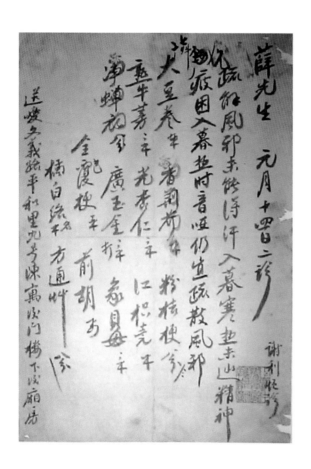

谢观处方

近现代

23 厘米 ×16 厘米

Prescription Written by Xie Guan

Modern Times

23 cm×16 cm

长方形，为处方，是谢观为薛先生所开处方，处方右下角有"谢利恒诊"字样，已装裱成册页。谢观（1880—1950）字利恒，江苏武进人，孟河名医，曾主持上海国医公会、中央国医馆等工作。其主编《中国医学大辞典》，反对废止中医案，著作较多，弟子甚众。保存基本完好。1962 年入藏。

中华医学会 / 上海中医药大学医史博物馆藏

This rectangular prescription was written by Xie Guan for Mr. Xue. There are characters "Xie Li Heng Zhen" on the lower right corner of the paper, which has been mounted in albums. Xie Guan (1880–1950), courtesy name Liheng, was born in Luo Shuwan, Wujin County, Jiangsu Province and was a famous doctor in Menghe Town. He was ever the head of Shanghai State Medical Association and Central Medical Hospital, and was the chief editor of *Grand Dictionary of Chinese Medicine*. He objected to the bill of abolishing Traditional Chinese Medicine. He compiled a lot of famous books, and had many students. This prescription was collected in 1962 and is well preserved.

Preserved in Chinese Medical Association/Museum of Chinese Medicine, Shanghai University of Traditional Chinese Medicine

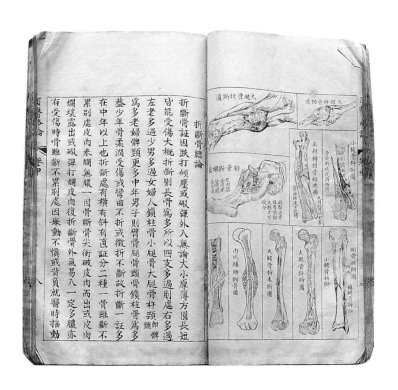

《西医略论》手抄本

近现代

28 厘米 ×18 厘米

上海仁济医院咸丰年间的出版物——《西医略论》手抄本。

上海医药文献博物馆藏

Manuscript of *A Brief Discussion on Western Medicine*

Modern Times

28 cm×18 cm

It was issued by Shanghai Renji Hospital during the reign of Emperor Xianfeng.

Preserved in Shanghai Medical Literature Museum

王仲奇处方

近现代

长 12.8 厘米，宽 7.5 厘米

王仲奇（1881－1945），名金杰，晚号懒翁，安徽歙县人，专精医术，擅医热病，对脏腑经络有较深研究，远近闻名，有"新安王氏医学"之称。此为其手书处方。

上海中医药博物馆藏

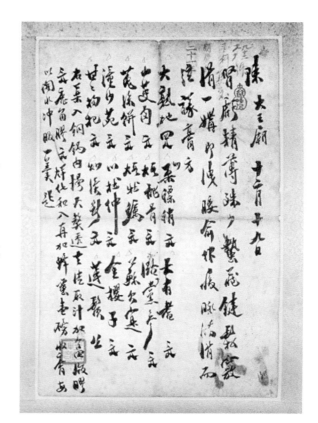

Prescription Written by Wang Zhongqi

Modern Times

Length 12.6 cm/ Width 7.5 cm

Wang Zhongqi (1881-1945), given name Jinjie, pseudonym name Lanweng, was born in Shexian County, Anhui Province. He was proficient in medical skill and good at treating fever disease. He was also famous for studying internal organs and meridians, and was known as "Doctor Wang of Xin'an". This is his hand-written prescription.

Preserved in Shanghai Museum of Traditional Chinese Medicine

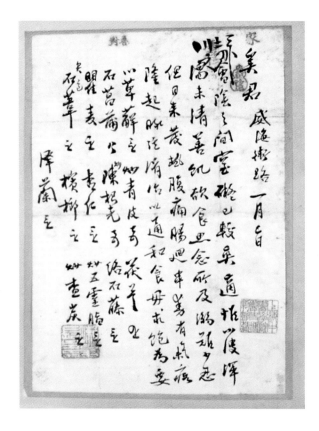

王仲奇处方

近现代

26 厘米 ×16.5 厘米

长方形，为处方。该藏用普通白纸写成，是王仲奇为奚君诊治小便浑浊、腹痛、发热等症所开处方之一，方末有"懒翁长寿"白文押记。保存基本完好。1960 年入藏。

中华医学会／上海中医药大学医史博物馆藏

Prescription Written by Wang Zhongqi

Modern Times

26 cm×16.5 cm

This rectangular prescription written on normal white paper was one of the prescriptions written by Wang Zhongqi for Xi Jun in treating the symptoms of disease, such as turbid urine, belly pain and fever. The end of this prescription was signed with an intaglio seal "Lan Wong Chang Shou". It was collected in 1960 and is well preserved.

Preserved in Chinese Medical Association/Museum of Chinese Medicine, Shanghai University of Traditional Chinese Medicine

王仲奇处方

近现代

25.8 厘米 ×16.5 厘米

长方形，为处方。该藏用普通白纸写成，是王仲奇为奚君诊治小便浑浊、腹痛、发热等症所开处方之一，方末有"懒翁长寿"白文押记。保存基本完好。1960 年入藏。

中华医学会 / 上海中医药大学医史博物馆藏

Prescription Written by Wang Zhongqi

Modern Times

25.8 cm×16.5 cm

This rectangular prescription written on normal white paper was one of the prescriptions written by Wang Zhongqi for Xi Jun in treating the symptoms of disease, such as turbid urine, belly pain and fever. The end of this prescription was signed with an intaglio seal "Lan Wong Chang Shou". It was collected in 1960 and is well preserved.

Preserved in Chinese Medical Association/Museum of Chinese Medicine, Shanghai University of Traditional Chinese Medicine

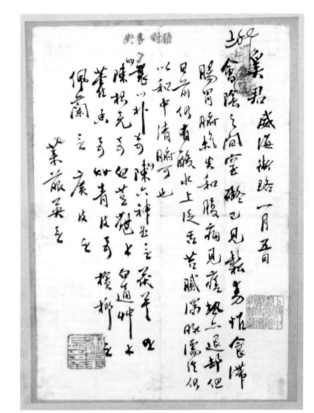

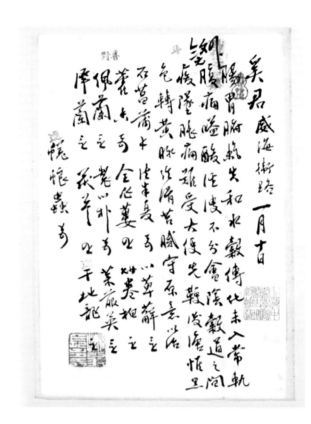

王仲奇处方

近现代

26 厘米 ×16.5 厘米

长方形，为处方。该藏用普通白纸写成，是王仲奇为奚君诊治小便浑浊、腹痛、发热等症所开处方之一，方末有"懒翁长寿"白文押记。保存基本完好。1960 年入藏。

中华医学会／上海中医药大学医史博物馆藏

Prescription Written by Wang Zhongqi

Modern Times

26 cm×16.5 cm

This rectangular prescription written on normal white paper was one of the prescriptions written by Wang Zhongqi for Xi Jun in treating the symptoms of disease, such as trubid urine, belly pain and fever. The end of this prescription was signed with an intaglio seal "Lan Wong Chang Shou". It was collected in 1960 and is well preserved.

Preserved in Chinese Medical Association/Museum of Chinese Medicine, Shanghai University of Traditional Chinese Medicine

王仲奇处方

近现代

26 厘米 ×16.5 厘米

长方形，为处方。该藏用普通白纸写成，是王仲奇为奚君诊治小便浑浊、腹痛、发热等症所开处方之一，方末有"懒翁长寿"白文押记。保存基本完好。1960 年入藏。

中华医学会 / 上海中医药大学医史博物馆藏

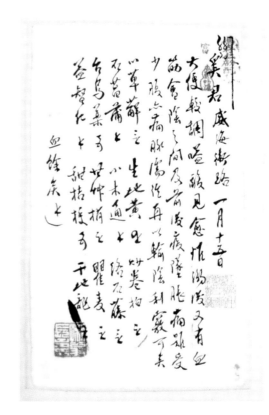

Prescription Written by Wang Zhongqi

Modern Times

26 cm×16.5 cm

This rectangular paper is a prescription. It was written on normal white paper, and was one of the prescriptions written by Wang Zhongqi for Xi Jun in treating the symptoms of disease, such as turbid urine, belly pain and fever. The end of this prescription was signed with a intaglio seal "Lan Wong Chang Shou". It is well preserved, and was collected in 1960.

Preserved in Chinese Medical Association/Museum of Chinese Medicine, Shanghai University of Traditional Chinese Medicine

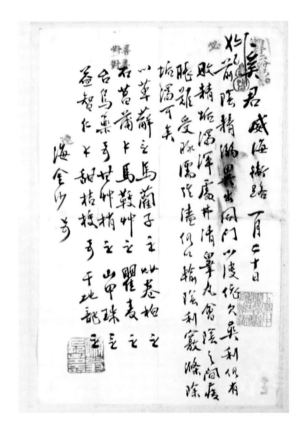

王仲奇处方

近现代

26 厘米 ×16.5 厘米

长方形，为处方。该藏用普通白纸写成，是王仲奇
为奚君诊治小便浑浊、腹痛、发热等症所开处方之
一，方末有"懒翁长寿"白文押记。保存基本完好。
1960 年入藏。

中华医学会 / 上海中医药大学医史博物馆藏

Prescription Written by Wang Zhongqi

Modern Times

26 cm×16.5 cm

This rectangular paper is a prescription. It was written
on normal white paper, and was one of the prescriptions
written by Wang Zhongqi for Xi Jun in treating the
symptoms of disease, such as turbid urine, belly pain
and fever. The end of this prescription was signed with
an intaglio seal "Lan Wong Chang Shou". It is well
preserved, and was collected in 1960.

Preserved in Chinese Medical Association/Museum of
Chinese Medicine, Shanghai University of Traditional
Chinese Medicine

王仲奇处方

近现代

26 厘米 ×16.5 厘米

长方形，为处方。该藏用普通白纸写成，是王仲奇为奚君诊治小便浑浊、腹痛、发热等症所开处方之一，方末有"懒翁长寿"白文押记。保存基本完好。1960 年入藏。

中华医学会 / 上海中医药大学医史博物馆藏

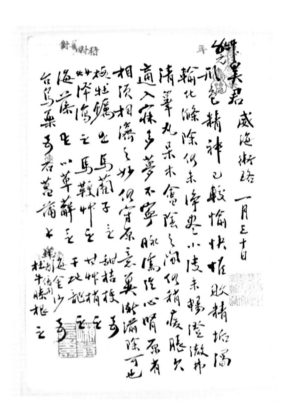

Prescription Written by Wang Zhongqi

Modern

Paper

26 cm×16.5 cm

This rectangular paper is a prescription. It was written on normal white paper, and was one of the prescriptions written by Wang Zhongqi for Xi Jun in treating the symptoms of disease, such as turbid urine, belly pain and fever. The end of this prescription was signed with a intaglio seal "Lan Wong Chang Shou". It is well preserved, and was collected in 1960.

Preserved in Chinese Medical Association/Museum of Chinese Medicine, Shanghai University of Traditional Chinese Medicine

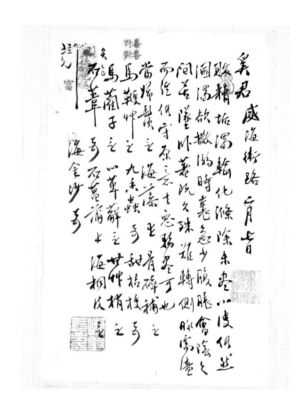

王仲奇处方

近现代

26 厘米 ×16.5 厘米

长方形，为处方。该藏用普通白纸写成，是王仲奇为奚君诊治小便浑浊、腹痛、发热等症所开处方之一，方末有"懒翁长寿"白文押记。保存基本完好。1960 年入藏。

中华医学会 / 上海中医药大学医史博物馆藏

Prescription Written by Wang Zhongqi

Modern Times

26 cm×16.5 cm

This rectangular paper is a prescription. It was written on normal white paper, and was one of the prescriptions written by Wang Zhongqi for Xi Jun in treating the symptomsof disease, such as turbid urine, belly pain and fever. The end of this prescription was signed with a intaglio seal "Lan Wong Chang Shou". It is well preserved, and was collected in 1960.

Preserved in Chinese Medical Association/Museum of Chinese Medicine, Shanghai University of Traditional Chinese Medicine

王仲奇处方

近现代

26 厘米 ×16.3 厘米

长方形，为处方。该藏用普通白纸写成，是王仲奇为奚君诊治小便浑浊、腹痛、发热等症所开处方之一，方末有"懒翁长寿"白文押记。保存基本完好。1960 年入藏。

中华医学会 / 上海中医药大学医史博物馆藏

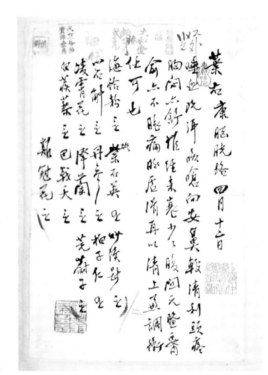

Prescription Written by Wang Zhongqi

Modern Times

26 cm×16.5 cm

This rectangular paper is a prescription. It was written on normal white paper, and was one of the prescriptions written by Wang Zhongqi for Xi Jun in treating the symptoms of disease, such as turbid urine, belly pain and fever. The end of this prescription was signed with an intaglio seal "Lan Wong Chang Shou". It is well preserved, and was collected in 1960.

Preserved in Chinese Medical Association/Museum of Chinese Medicine, Shanghai University of Traditional Chinese Medicine

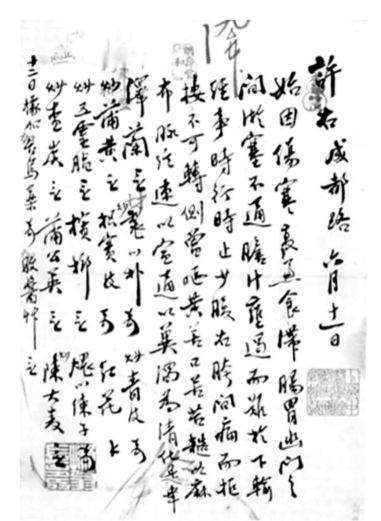

王仲奇处方

近现代

26 厘米 ×16.5 厘米

Prescription Written by Wang Zhongqi

Modern Times

26 cm×16.5 cm

长方形，为处方。该藏用普通白纸写成，是
王仲奇为许女士诊治伤寒高热食滞肠胃淤塞
胆汁壅遏等症所开处方之一，方末有"懒翁
长寿"白文押记。保存基本完好。1960 年
入藏。

中华医学会 / 上海中医药大学医史博物馆藏

This rectangular paper is a prescription. It was
written on normal white paper, and was one of
the prescriptions written by Wang Zhongqi for
Ms. Xu in treating the symptoms of disease,
such as typhoid fever, high fever, dyspepsia
and bile obstruction. The end of this
prescription was signed with an intaglio seal
"Lan Wong Chang Shou". This prescription is
well preserved, and was collected in 1960.
Preserved in Chinese Medical Association/
Museum of Chinese Medicine, Shanghai
University of Traditional Chinese Medicine

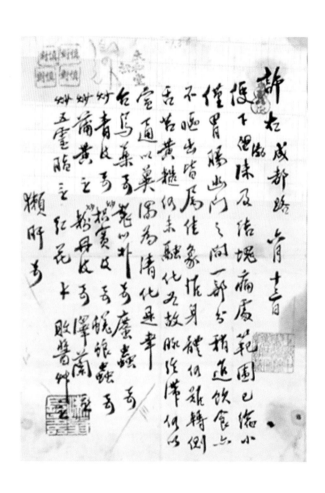

王仲奇处方

近现代

26 厘米 ×16.5 厘米

Prescription Written by Wang Zhongqi

Modern

26 cm×16.5 cm

长方形，为处方。该藏用普通白纸写成，是
王仲奇为许女士诊治伤寒高热食滞肠胃淤塞
胆汁壅遏等症所开处方之一，方末有"懒翁
长寿"白文押记。保存基本完好。1960年入藏。

中华医学会 / 上海中医药大学医史博物馆藏

This rectangular paper is a prescription. It was
written on normal white paper, and was one of
the prescriptions written by Wang Zhongqi for
Ms. Xu in treating the symptoms of disease,
such as typhoid fever,high fever, dyspepsia and
bile obstruction. The end of this prescription
was signed with an intaglio seal "Lan Wong
Chang Shou". This prescription is well
preserved, and was collected in 1960.

Preserved in Chinese Medical Association/
Museum of Chinese Medicine, Shanghai
University of Traditional Chinese Medicine

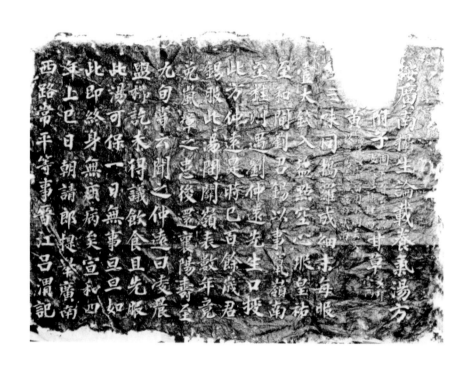

养气汤方拓片

近现代

石刻片：长 66 厘米，宽 43 厘米

真书：长 2.8 厘米，宽 1.4 厘米

Rubbing of Yang Qi Tang Fang

Modern Times

Stone Cutting: 66 cm×43 cm

Character: 2.8: cm×1.4 cm

原刻为近现代桂林南溪山刘仙岩上之摩崖石刻。

上题"宣和四年（1122）朝请郎提举广南西路

常平等事、晋江吕渭记"字样。

北京中医药大学中医药博物馆藏

The inscription "Yang Qi Tang Fang" (Recipes for Promoting Qi) was originally carved on Liu Xian Cliff, Nan Xi Mountain in Guilin City. On the rubbing are characters recording the history of the stone inscription in 1122.

Preserved in The Museum of Chinese Medicine, Beijing University of Chinese Medicine

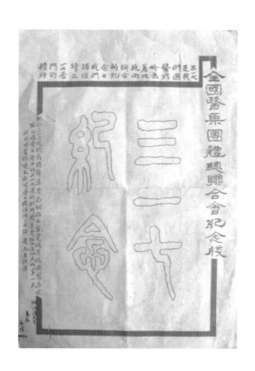

便笺

近现代

长 29.5 厘米，宽 21 厘米

全国医药团体总联合会"三一七"纪念笺。

江苏省中医药博物馆藏

Notepaper Memo

Modern Times

Length 29.5 cm/ Width 21 cm

This is a memorial notepaper for the 'March 17th Incident' (the abolition bill of Traditional Chinese Medicine in 1929) of The National Association of Medical Organizations.

Preserved in Jiangsu Museum of Traditional Chinese Medicine

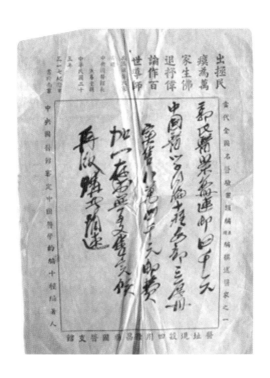

便笺

近现代

长 26.8 厘米，宽 19 厘米

中央国医馆便笺。

江苏省中医药博物馆藏

Notepaper Memo

Modern Times

Length 26.8 cm/ Width 19 cm

This is a notepaper memo of the National Traditional Chinese Medical Center.

Preserved in Jiangsu Museum of Traditional Chinese Medicine

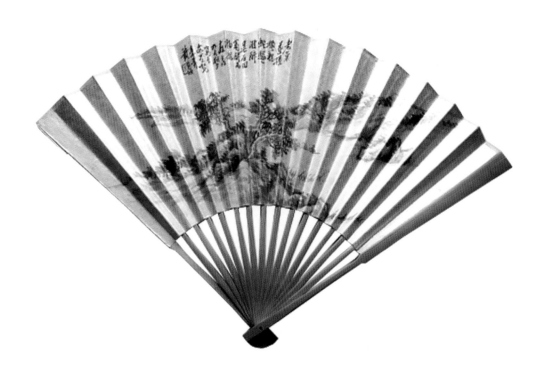

陆渊雷书画扇

近现代

扇长 32.2 厘米，扇面上宽 50.5 厘米，下宽 21.5 厘米，高 18.3 厘米

Calligraphy and Painting on Fan by Lu Yuanlei

Modern Times

Length 32.2 cm/ Upper Width of the Fan Face 50.5 cm/ Lower Width 21.5 cm/ Height 18.3 cm

扇状，是艺术品。该藏是民国十八年（1929）初秋陆渊雷所作，扇面一面为山水国画，另面为篆书骈文，共48字，题赠文荃先生。陆渊雷(1894－1955)，字彭年，江苏川沙（今上海浦东）人，医家。1929年与徐衡之创办上海国医学院，后任中央国医馆学术委员，创刊《中医新生命》杂志，学以中西医汇通著称。已装裱成镜片，保存基本完好。1957年入藏。

中华医学会 / 上海中医药大学医史博物馆藏

This piece of artwork is in the shape of a fan, which was made by Lu Yuanlei in early autumn of 1929 (the 18th year of the Republic of China). One side of the fan face is designed with Chinese landscape painting, and the other side is inscribed with a parallel prose of forty-eight words written in seal character which is dedicated to Mr. Wen Quan. Lu Yuanlei (1894–1955), courtesy name Peng Nian, was from Chuansha County in Jiangsu Province(now as Pudong District in Shanghai). He was a physician famous for his integration of both Chinese Medicine and Western Medicine. In 1929, he established the Shanghai School of Chinese Medicine together with Xu Hengzhi. Later, he served as the academic committee member of the National Traditional Chinese Medical Center and founded the journal "Zhong Yi Xin Sheng Ming" (*New Life of Traditional Chinese Medicine*). This piece of artwork has been framed and is preserved well. It was collected in 1957

Preserved in Chinese Medical Association/Museum of Chinese Medicine, Shanghai University of Traditional Chinese Medicine

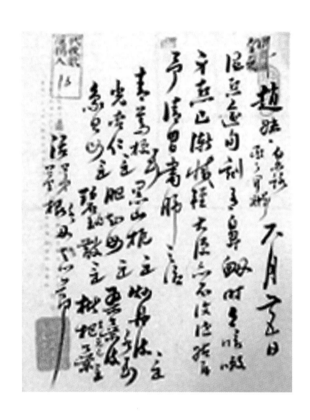

严苍山亲笔处方

近现代

处方：长 26 厘米，宽 18.6 厘米

镜片：40 厘米 ×31.3 厘米

Handwritten Prescription by Yan Cangshan

Modern Times

Length 26 cm/ Width 18.6 cm

The framed Glass: 40 cm×31.3 cm

镜片，为处方。该处方为严氏于1942年后在法租界莆柏路、贝勒路口420号寓中为赵妹所开处方。有白文"宁海医家严苍山氏壬午后处方之记"草绿押记，并印有"门人郑衡若、翁韻竹、侄世英、张利彬、居澹秋、陈雲帆侍诊"字样。严苍山（1898—1968）名云，浙江宁海人，从祖习医，1927年参与创办中国医学院，1932年被聘为中国国医馆发起人。中华人民共和国成立后，其组织卢湾区第二联合诊所，任上海中医学会常委兼秘书长、市政协委员等职。严氏精通医典，善治急症、重症，著有《疫痉家庭自疗集》《汤头歌诀续集》等。处方已装裱成镜片，保存基本完好。1997年入藏。

中华医学会 / 上海中医药大学医史博物馆藏

This prescription is made into a frame. It was prescribed for Zhaomei by Yan at his residence in No.420 Baylor Road, Pubai Road of French Concession after 1942. There was a green pledge with intagliated characters meaning "prescribed by Yan Cangshan from Ninghai County in the year of Renwu" and the printed characters meaning "disciples of Zheng Hengruo, Weng Yunzhu, Zhi Shiying, Zhang Libin, Ju Danqiu and Chen Yunfan attended the diagnosis ". Yan cangshan (1898–1968), with the given name of Yun, was from Ninghai County of Zhejiang Province. He learned medicine from his forefathers and participated in the establishment of China's School of Medicine in 1927. In 1932, He was appointed as the initiator of National Traditional Chinese Medical Center. After liberation, he established the second polyclinic at Luwan District and served as member of the standing committee and general-secretary of Shanghai Academy of Chinese Medicine, and member of the Municipal Political Consultative Conference. Yan was proficient in medical Knowledge and was good at treatming acute and severe symptoms. He wrote the medical book of *Yi Jing Jia Ting Zi Liao Ji* (collection of family therapy in treating epidemic disease and spasm) and *Tang Tou Ge Jue Xu Ji* (sequel of recipe of decoction written in verse). The preseription has been framed and is preserved well. It was collected in 1997.

Preserved in Chinese Medical Association/Museum of Chinese Medicine, Shanghai University of Traditional Chinese Medicine

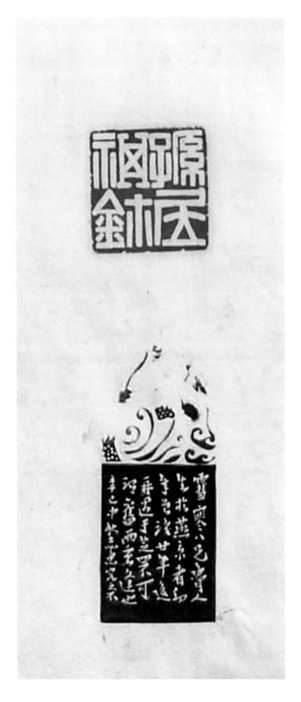

印谱

近现代

长 23 厘米，宽 12.6 厘米

Collection of Seal Designs

Modern Times

Length 23 cm/ Width 12.6 cm

纸张形，为印谱，为线装本，兰色封皮。书内序、跋皆无，编者、年代均不详，全书共96页。印谱装帧较讲究，保存完好。

中华医学会 / 上海中医药大学医史博物馆藏

This is a paper collection of seal stamps. It is a thread-bound edition with blue covers. The book has ninety-six pages without preface or postscript, nor the author and the time. It was of good binding and layout and is preserved well. Preserved in Chinese Medical Association/ Museum of Chinese Medicine, Shanghai University of Traditional Chinese Medicine

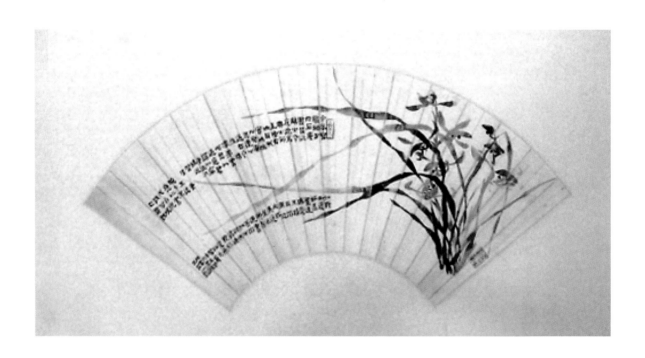

程门雪墨兰扇面

近现代

扇面上宽 50 厘米，下宽 21 厘米，高 17.9 厘米

Painting of Chinese Cymbidium on Fan by Cheng Menxue

Modern Times

Upper Width of the Fan Face 50 cm/ Lower Width 21cm/ Height 17.9 cm

镜片，为艺术品，系程门雪于 1941 年所绘，赠于门生徐培泽，以勉励他钻研学问。落款"门雪"并钤白文朱印。扇面右下钤篆体朱文"何氏二十八世医藏"印。程门雪（1902—1972），名振辉，号九如、壶公，婺源人，幼小从师名医汪莲石、丁甘仁习医。1956 年任上海中医学院（今上海中医药大学）首任院长，是近现代中医名家。已装裱成镜片，保存基本完好。1991 年入藏。

中华医学会 / 上海中医药大学医史博物馆藏

This framed piece of artwork was painted by Cheng Menxue in 1941. He gave it to his disciple Xu Peize as a gift to encourage him to endeavor to study. The badging is inscribed with characters of "Men Xue" and an official intaglio seal. The lower right side of the fan face is inscribed with the relief seal saying "preserved by the twenty eighth physicians of the Family He". Cheng Menxue (1902–1972), given name Zhen Hui, pseudonym Jiu Ru and Hu Gong, was from Wuyuan County, Jiangxi Province. He learned from the famous physician Wang Lianshi and Ding Ganren when he was a child. He was a famous Traditional Chinese Medicine physician in modern times and was the first dean of Shanghai College of Traditional Chinese Medicine (now as Shanghai University of Traditional Chinese Medicine) in 1956. The fan has been framed and is preserved well. It was collected in 1991. Preserved in Chinese Medical Association/Museum of Chinese Medicine, Shanghai University of Traditional Chinese Medicine

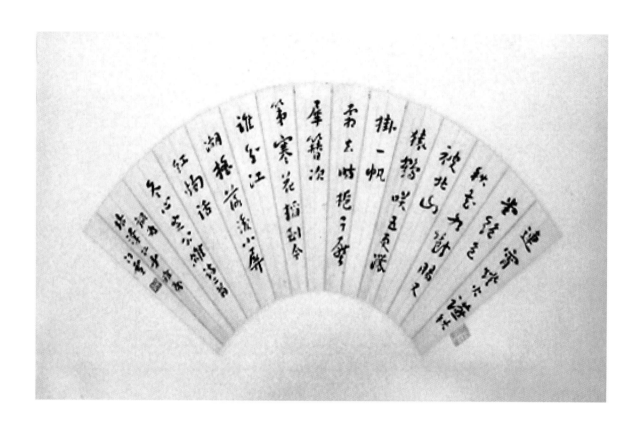

程门雪"冬心诗"书扇面

近现代

扇面上宽 50 厘米，下宽 21.3 厘米，高 17.8 厘米

Calligraphy of "Dong Xin" Poem by Cheng Menxue

Modern Times

Upper Width of the Fan Face 50 cm/ Lower Width 21.3 cm/ Height 17.8 cm

镜片，为艺术品，系程门雪书冬心杂诗二首。题
赠"培泽仁弟"。落款"门雪"并钤白文朱印。
镜片右下钤篆体朱文"何氏二十八世医藏"印。
已装裱成镜片，保存基本完好。1991年入藏。

中华医学会 / 上海中医药大学医史博物馆藏

This framed piece of artwork was painted by Cheng
Menxue with two poems named "Dong Xin". He
gave it to his disciple Xu Peize as a gift. The
badging is inscribed with characters of "Men Xue"
and an official intaglio seal. The lower right side
of the fan face is inscribed with the relief seal "He
Shi Er Shi Ba Shi Yi Cang" saying "preserved by
the twenty eighth physician of the Family He". The
fan has been framed and is preserved well. It was
collected in 1991.
Preserved in Chinese Medical Association/Museum
of Chinese Medicine, Shanghai University of
Traditional Chinese Medicine

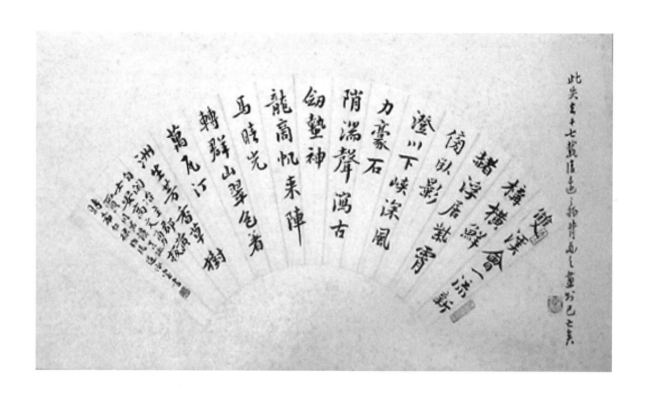

道依室临蔡君漠扇面

近现代

扇面：上宽 51.5 厘米，下宽 22.9 厘米，高 17.7 厘米

镜片：长 61.5 厘米，宽 32.7 厘米

Facsimile of Cai Junmo's Calligraphy on Fan by Dao Yishi

Modern Times

Upper: Width 51.5 cm/ Lower Width 22.9 cm/ Height 17.7 cm

Frame: Length 61.5 cm/ Width 32.7 cm

扇状，为艺术品，为道依室（可能为程门雪的别号）临蔡君漠扇面。题赠"时希仁棣雅玩"，落款"道依室书"并朱印记四方，其中两方为何时希白文印记，一方为程门雪朱文"壶公"押记，另一方待考。镜片左端有何时希书"此失去十七载复还之物面之画则已亡矣"。已装裱成镜片，保存基本完好。1991 年入藏。

中华医学会 / 上海中医药大学医史博物馆藏

This piece of artwork is in the shape of a fan. It was a piece of Dao Yishi's (maybe a pseudonym of Cheng Menxue) fan artwork with imitations of Cai Junmo's calligraphy work. There are inscriptions of the characters "Shi Xi Ren Di Ya Wan" (indicating the receiver of the gift) and a badging of "written by Daoyishi" inscribed with four red seals. Two of them are He Shixi's (a famous physician) seals of intagliated characters. One is Cheng Menxue's seal with characters "Hu Gong" cut in relief. The fourth one remains unverified. The left part of the piece is inscribed with He Shixi's words of "this piece of artwork had been lost for seventeen years, and the painting on it had been destroyed after its regaining ". It has been framed and is preserved well. It was collected in 1991. Preserved in Chinese Medical Association/Museum of Chinese Medicine, Shanghai University of Traditional Chinese Medicine

程师诗书画集葺成记后

近现代

画芯长 30.3 厘米，宽 21.5 厘米

镜片，为艺术品，为程门雪学生何时希"《程门雪诗书画集》葺成记后"楷书手稿。已装裱成镜片，保存基本完好。1991 年入藏。

中华医学会 / 上海中医药大学医史博物馆藏

Postscript on Repairing Teacher Cheng's Works

Modern

Length 30.3 cm/ Width 21.5 cm (without margin)

This piece of artwork is framed. It was a manuscript of He Shixi who was Cheng Menxue's student. It was written in seal character as a postscript on repairing *Cheng Menxue Shi Shu Hua Ji* (Cheng's work collection with poems, paintings and calligraphy works). It is preserved well. It was collected in 1991.

Preserved in Chinese Medical Association/Museum of Chinese Medicine, Shanghai University of Traditional Chinese Medicine

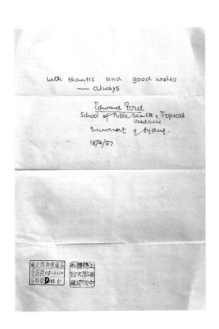

EDWARD FORD 贺词

近现代（1957）

25.7 厘米 ×17.7 厘米

长方形，为贺词，普通信纸书就，是 1957 年 4 月
18 日 Edward Ford 亲笔贺辞，具体内容为 "With
thanks and good wishes —always"，并亲笔
签名和属 "Shool of Public Health & Tropical
Medicine" 和 "Sydny" 等字样。保存完好。
1958 年入藏。

中华医学会 / 上海中医药大学医史博物馆藏

Letter of Congratulations From Edward Ford

Modern Times (1957)

25.7 cm×17.7 cm

This is a letter of congratulations in rectangular
shape. It was written on an ordinary letter paper.
The congratulation letter is Edward Ford's own
handwriting on April 18th , 1957. The content of
the letter goes like this:"With thanks and good
wishes–always" and together with his signature
and the words "Shool of Public Health & Tropical
Medicine " and "Sydny". It was collected in 1958
and is preserved well.

Preserved in Chinese Medical Association/Museum
of Chinese Medicine, Shanghai University of
Traditional Chinese Medicine

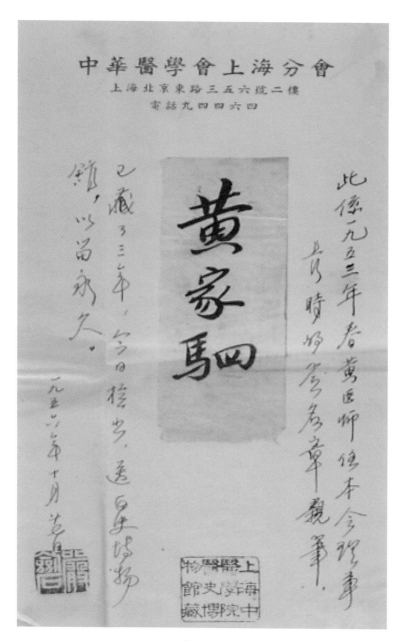

"黄家驷"签字式

近现代

9.8 厘米 ×3.6 厘米

Signature of Huang Jiasi

Modern Times

9.8 cm×3.6 cm

长方形，为签名。该签名粘贴于中华医学会上海分会便笺纸上，便笺上有严剑石注释，说明该签名为 1953 年春黄氏任本会理事长时的亲笔签名。黄家驷，江西人，1933 年毕业于北京协和医学院，获医学博士，我国胸腔外科奠基人之一，在国内外医界有广泛的联系和影响。保存完好。1958 年入藏。

中华医学会 / 上海中医药大学医史博物馆藏

This is a piece of signature in rectangular shape. It was pasted on the notepaper of Shanghai branch of Chinese Medical Association. On the notepaper, there is an explanatory note written by Yan Jianshi which proved that this is the autograph of Huang Jiasi signed in spring of 1953 when he served as the director general of the association. Huang Jiasi, a native of Jiangxi Province, graduated from Peking Union Medical College in 1933 and received the degree of Doctor of Medicine. He was one of the founders in thoracic surgery in our country. He had extensive contacts and wide influences in both home and abroad. It was collected in 1958 and is preserved well.

Preserved in Chinese Medical Association/Museum of Chinese Medicine, Shanghai University of Traditional Chinese Medicine

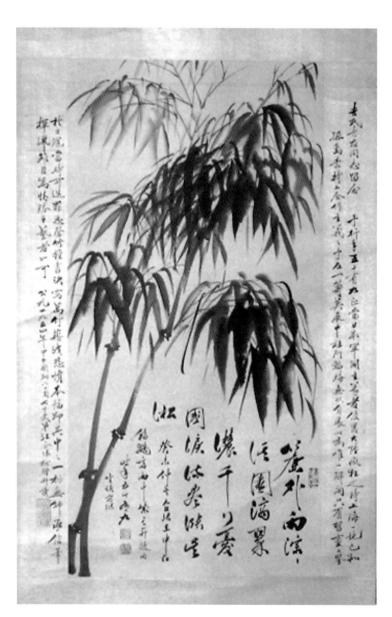

汪企张画竹图

近现代

画芯：长 67 厘米，宽 31.2 厘米

卷轴：长 188 厘米，宽 44.8 厘米

Painting of Bamboo by Wang Qizhang

Modern Times

Painting: Length 67 cm/ Width 31.2 cm

Scroll: Length 188 cm/ Width 44.8 cm

卷轴，为书画。汪企张所绘。画面为汪企张于 1943 年
59 岁画的墨竹，时值日寇入侵，罪恶罄竹难书，因画竹
以表愤怒。画外注明该画于 1954 年在甲午国耻 60 周年
之际赠与王吉民，是年汪企张已 70 岁。已裱成卷轴，纸
张泛黄，画面有污迹。

中华医学会 / 上海中医药大学医史博物馆藏

This piece of artwork is a scroll with calligraphy and
painting. It is an ink painting of bamboo painted by Wang
Qizhang when he was fifty-nine years old in 1943. At that
time, China was invaded by the Japanese Army which had
committed countless crimes in China. As a result, Wang
painted bamboos to express his anger. It was indicated
outside the painting that this bamboo painting was given
to Wang Jimin as a gift in 1954 when it was the 60th
anniversary of the Sino-Japanese war of 1894–1895, and
Wang Qizhang was seventy years old then. It has been
framed into scroll and the paper is yellowing and with stains
in the picture.

Preserved in Chinese Medical Association/Museum of
Chinese Medicine, Shanghai University of Traditional
Chinese Medicine

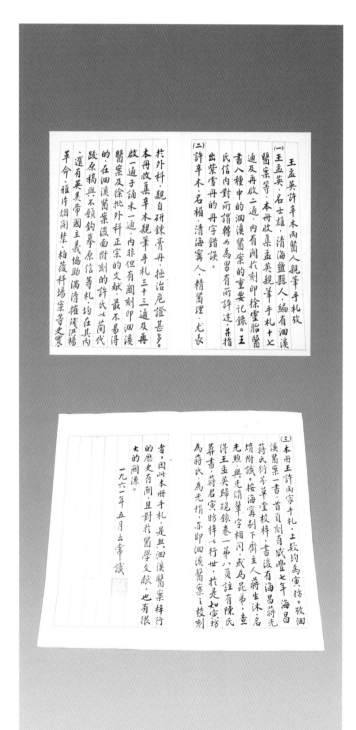

云常笔札

近现代

39.5 厘米 ×36 厘米

Yun Chang's Writing Materials

Modern Times

39.5 cm×36 cm

长方形，为手稿。该藏白纸墨书对折。该笔札
为 1961 年 5 月写就，是云常笔札的后半部分，
内容关于王孟英、许辛木两医师的情况。保存
基本完好。1961 年入藏。

中华医学会 / 上海中医药大学医史博物馆藏

This is a manuscript of rectangular shape. It is
in folio form with ink characters on the white
paper. Here is the latter half of the materials. This
writing material was finished in May 1961, and
some introductions of the two physicians Wang
Mengying and Xu Xinmu were included. It was
collected in 1958 and is preserved well.
Preserved in Chinese Medical Association/
Museum of Chinese Medicine, Shanghai
University of Traditional Chinese Medicine

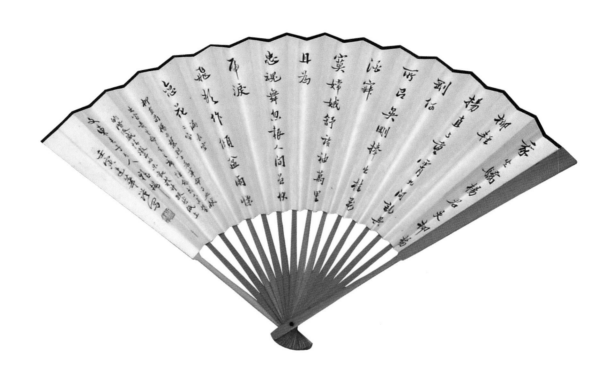

徐嵩年赠黄文东书画扇

近现代

扇长 30.1 厘米 ，扇面上宽 45.5 厘米，下宽 17.6 厘米，高 30 厘米

Fan with Calligraphy Presented by Xu Songnian to Huang Wendong

Modern Times

Length 30.1 cm/ Upper Width of the Fan Face 45.5 cm/ Lower Width 17.6 cm/ Height 30 cm

扇状，是艺术品。该藏是 1962 年徐嵩年、胡建华赠给
老师黄文东先生的书画扇。扇面一面为人物山水画（徐
嵩年画），题赠"文东夫子大人"，并落款"嵩年"及
钤朱文押记。另面为胡建华行楷毛主席诗词《蝶恋花》，
且于词末书该词相关注释及落款钤印。徐嵩年和胡建
华是黄文东的学生。已装裱成镜片，保存基本完好。
1997 年入藏。

中华医学会 / 上海中医药大学医史博物馆藏

This piece of artwork is in the shape of a fan, which was
presented by Xu Songnian and Hu Jianhua to their teacher
Huang Wendong. One side of the fan face is decorated
with a painting of people and landscape (painted by Xu
Songnian), inscription of "Dear teacher Wendong "and
a badging of "Songnian" with an official relief seal. The
other side of the fan is the inscription of Chairman Mao's
poem "Die Lian Hua" (*Love of Butterfly*) written in seal
character by Hu Jianhua, and at the end of the poem is the
related annotation about the poem as well as the badging and
official seal. Xu Songnian and Hu Jianhua were students of
Huang Wendong. This piece of artwork has been framed and
is preserved well. It was collected in 1997.
Preserved in Chinese Medical Association/Museum of
Chinese Medicine, Shanghai University of Traditional
Chinese Medicine

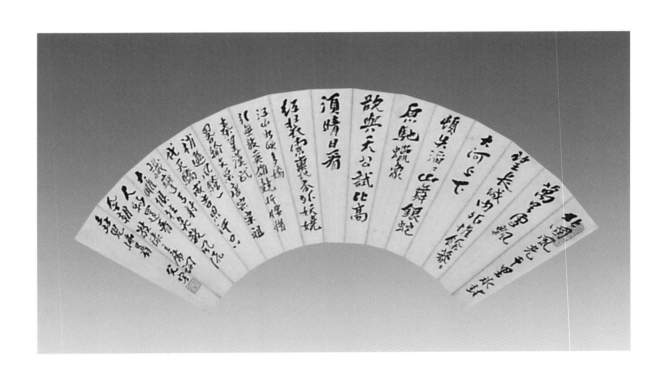

陆瘦燕书扇面

近现代

扇面：上宽 42.5 厘米，下宽 20.3 厘米，高 12.9 厘米

镜片：66.7 厘米 ×39.8 厘米

Fan Face with Lu Shouyan's Calligraphy Work

Modern Times

Fan: Upper Width 42.5 cm/ Lower Width 20.3 cm/ Height 12.9 cm

Frame: 66.7 cm×39.8 cm

镜片，是艺术品。该藏是陆瘦燕书毛泽东词《沁园春·雪》赠爱女陆焱垚的扇面。1996 年为庆祝上海中医药大学建校 40 周年陆焱垚捐赠我馆。陆瘦燕（1909—1969），本名李名昌，原籍嘉定，后出嗣陆家，寄籍昆山。自幼随父习医，1948 年兴办新中国针灸学研究社，影响远及东南亚。主要论著有《针灸正宗》《经络学图说》《针灸法汇论》《腧穴学概论》等。另有夫人及门人整理出版《陆瘦燕针灸论著医案选》。已装裱成镜片，保存基本完好。1997 年入藏。

中华医学会 / 上海中医药大学医史博物馆藏

This piece of calligraphy work of Mao Zedong's peom *Qin Yuan Chun-Xue* was written by Lu Shouyan for his daughter Lu Yanyao, who then donated it to the museum in 1996 in celebration of 40th anniversary of the establishment of Shanghai University of Traditional Chinese Medicine. Lu Shouyan (1909–1969), with an original name of Li Mingchang born in Jiading County, was later given to the family of Lu as their son and lived in Kunshan County. He learned Chinese Medicine from his father when he was a child and established China's Acupuncture Research Institute in 1948, which had a great influence even on the Southeast Asian countries. His main masterpieces are *Zhen Jiu Zheng Zong* (Acupuncture and Moxibustion), *Jing Luo Xue Tu Shuo* (an illustration of collaterals), *Zhen Jiu Fa Hui Lun* (a collection of methods for acupuncture and moxibustion), and *Shu Xue Xue Gai Lun* (introduction on the knowledge of acupoints). There is also the book *Collection of Lu Shouyan's Medical Record on Acupuncture and Moxibustion*, which was composed and published by his wife and disciples. This fan face has been framed and is preserved well. It was collected in 1997.

Preserved in Chinese Medical Association/Museum of Chinese Medicine, Shanghai University of Traditional Chinese Medicine

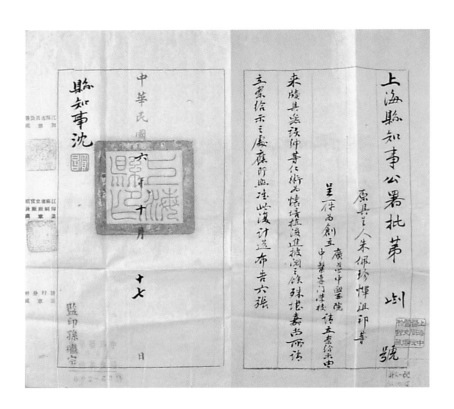

上海广益中医院、上海中医专门学校成立批文

近现代

30.9 厘米 ×26.5 厘米

Approval Document of Shanghai Guangyi TCM Hospital and Shanghai TCM Specialized School

Modern Times

30.9 cm×26.5 cm

长方形，为批文，是民国六年十月十七日上海县知事公署批准创立"上海市广益中医院、上海中医专门学校"的文书，文末钤"上海县印"并县知事沈宝昌押记，还钤江苏省长公署和江苏省官纸印刷厂厂长等印鉴。保存完好。1955年入藏。

中华医学会 / 上海中医药大学医史博物馆藏

This rectangle document was an approval authorized by Shanghai County Government Office on October 17, the sixth year of Republic of China for the establishment of "Shanghai Guangyi Traditional Chinese Medicine Hospital and Shanghai Traditional Chinese Medicine Specialize School". At the end of the document was affixed an official seal of "Shanghai Xian Yin (Shanghai County seal)" with the charge of Shen Baochang, magistrate of the County, as well as seals of Jiangsu provincial governors' office and manager of official paper print house of Jiangsu Province, etc. The approval is well preserved. It was collected in 1955. Preserved in Chinese Medical Association/Museum of Chinese Medicine, Shanghai University of Traditional Chinese Medicine

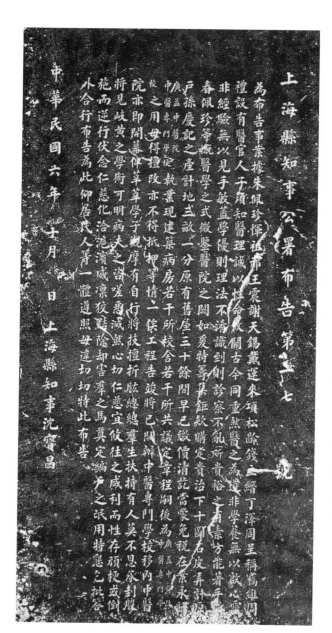

上海县知事公署布告（278 号）拓片

近现代

长 136 厘米，宽 67.7 厘米

1917 年为建立广益中医院并中医专门学校，上海知事沈宝昌特发布告，立碑记事。

上海中医药博物馆藏

Rubbing of Shanghai County Government Notice (No. 278)

Modern Times

Length 136cm/ Width 67.7cm

In 1917, in order to establish Guangyi Traditional Chinese Medicine Hospital and Traditional Chinese Medicine Specialized School, Shen Baochang, magistrate of Shanghai County, specially put this notice up and set up a monument to record the event.

Preserved in Shanghai Museum of Traditional Chinese Medicine

上海沪南广益中医院并中医专门学校碑记拓片

近现代

长 135 厘米，宽 65 厘米

1918 年，上海沪南广益中医院并中医专门学校建立时所立碑拓片。

上海中医药博物馆藏

Rubbing of Inscriptional Record of Guangyi TCM Hospital and TCM Specialized School in Southern Shanghai

Modern Times

Length 135 cm/ Width 65 cm

It is the rubbing of the stele that was set up in 1918 when Guangyi Traditional Chinese Medicine Hospital and Traditional Chinese Medicine Specialized School in southern Shanghai were established.

Preserved in Shanghai Museum of Traditional Chinese Medicine

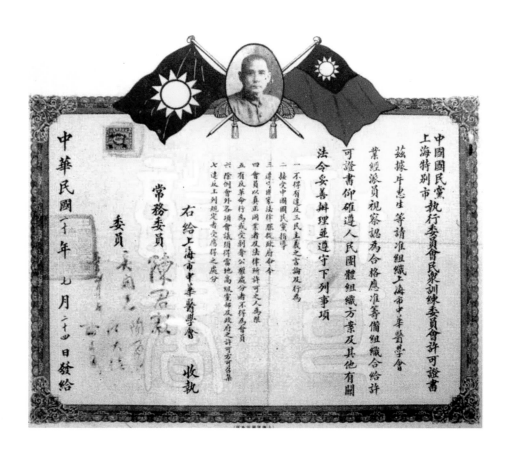

组织成立中华医学会许可证书

近现代

45 厘米 ×34.5 厘米

Approval Certificate of the Foundation of the Chinese Medical Association

Modern Times

45 cm×34.5 cm

中华医学会1915年在上海成立，主要从事医学
著作的编辑、翻译，医学教育的研究，名词审定，
医学标准的拟订等学术活动及会员的福利工作。
此为国民政府颁发的许可证书。

上海中医药博物馆藏

The Chinese Medical Association was founded
in Shanghai in 1915. It mainly worked on editing
and translating medical works, researching on
medical education, checking terminologies, drafting
medical criteria and other academic activities as
well as the welfare issues of the members. This
was the approval certificate issued by the national
government.

Preserved in Shanghai Museum of Traditional
Chinese Medicine

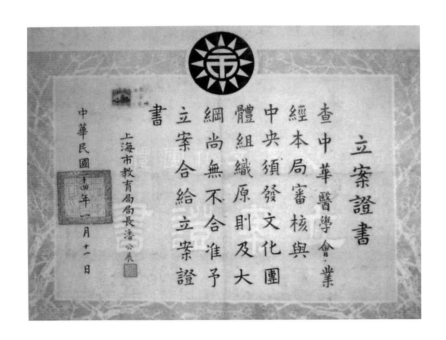

上海市教育局立案证书

近现代

48.5 厘米 ×37 厘米

长方形，为许可证。该藏为民国 24 年 1 月 11 日上海市教育局审核中华医学会文化团体组织资格合格准予立案的立案证书。保存基本完好。1953 年入藏。

中华医学会 / 上海中医药大学医史博物馆藏

Register Certificate by Shanghai Education Bureau

Modern Times

48.5 cm×37 cm

The rectangular register certificate was issued by Shanghai Education Bureau on January 11, the 24th year of the Republic of China, to grant the register of the Chinese Medical Association, a cultural organization qualified after examination and verification. It is basically well preserved. The certificate was collected in 1953.

Preserved in Chinese Medical Association/Museum of Chinese Medicine, Shanghai University of Traditional Chinese Medicine

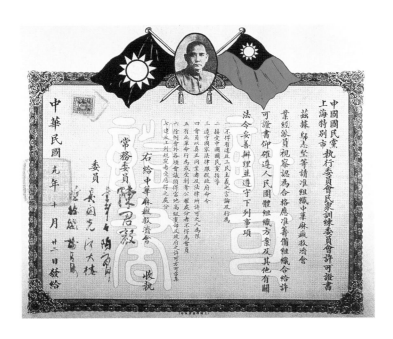

"中国麻风救济会" 筹组许可证书

近现代

47 厘米 ×36 厘米

此为 1930 年中国国民党上海特别市执行委员会民众训练委员会所颁发准许由邬志坚等人筹组 "中国麻风救济会" 的许可证书。

上海中医药博物馆藏

Approval Centificate for "Chinese Mission to Leprosy"

Modern Times

47 cm×36 cm

This certificate was issued by the Public Training Committee of Nationalist Party of China Executive Committee of Shanghai Special City in 1930, which permitted the preparation and organization of "Chinese Mission to Leprosy" by Wu Zhijian and others.

Preserved in Shanghai Museum of Traditional Chinese Medicine

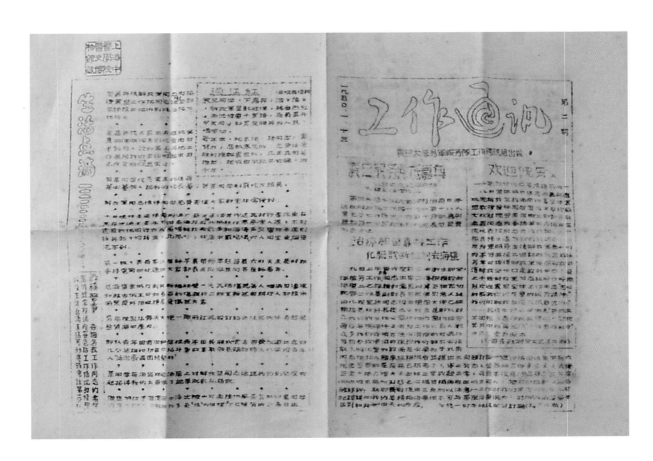

震旦大学为军服务队工作通讯

近现代

38.2 厘米 ×26.6 厘米

The Work Flyer of Aurora University's Service Team for the Army

Modern Times

38.2 cm×26.6 cm

长方形，宣传用。该藏用普通白纸油印，对折，为 1950 年日本住血吸虫肆虐期间震旦大学师生为人民解放军医疗治病服务队的工作通讯。保存基本完好。1955 年入藏。

中华医学会 / 上海中医药大学医史博物馆藏

The work flyer in rectangle shape was used for publicity. This collection was mimeographed in ordinary white paper in folio. It was the work flyer of the service team organized by teachers and students in Aurora University which provided medical treatments for the People's Liberation Army during the raging of Schistosoma japonicum in 1950. It is basically well preserved. It was collected in 1955. Preserved in Chinese Medical Association/ Museum of Chinese Medicine, Shanghai University of Traditional Chinese Medicine

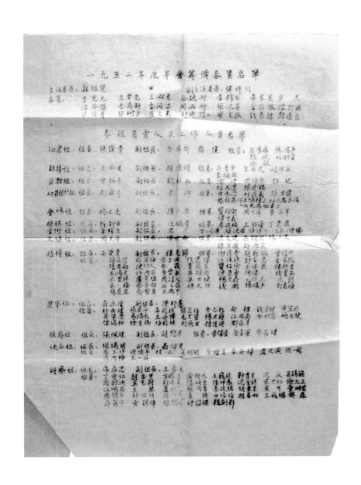

1952 年度年会筹备委员名单

近现代

35 厘米 ×25.3 厘米

The Name List of the Annual Meeting Preparatory Committee in 1952

Modern Times

35 cm×25.3 cm

长方形，为会议计划。该藏为普通白纸油印，为 1952 年度上海医师公会年会筹备委员名单，其主任委员为苏祖斐，副主任委员侯祥川，委员 21 人，并有年会秘书组、财务组、宣教组、动员组织组、会场组、联络组、学术组、文艺组、招待组、选举组、服务组、供应组、纠察组共 13 组的组长、副组长和组员名单。保存基本完好。1955 年入藏。

中华医学会 / 上海中医药大学医史博物馆藏

This meeting plan is in rectangle shape and was mimeographed in ordinary white paper. It records names of members in the Annual Meeting Preparatory Committee in 1952, which included Su Zufei, Chairman of the Committee; Hou Xiangchuan, vice-Chairman of the Committee; 21 committee members as well as group leaders; vice group leaders and group members of 13 groups, that is, annual meeting's secretary group, financing group, propaganda and education group, mobilization and organization group, meeting place group, contact group, academic group, art group, reception group, election group, service group, supply group and picket group. It is basically well preserved. It was collected in 1955.
Preserved in Chinese Medical Association/Museum of Chinese Medicine, Shanghai University of Traditional Chinese Medicine

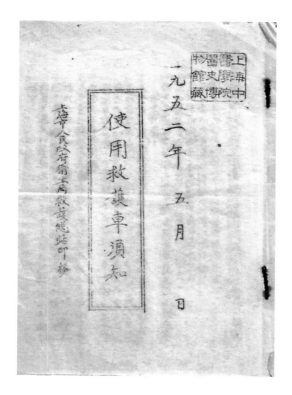

使用救护车须知

近现代

15.8 厘米 ×11.2 厘米

长方形，为工作须知。普通白纸竖排油印装订成册，内容分十条并公布各救护分站负责范围及联系电话，由上海市人民政府卫生局救护总站印发。保存完好。1955 年入藏。

中华医学会 / 上海中医药大学医史博物馆藏

The Instruction for Use of Ambulances

Modern Times

15.8 cm×11.2 cm

This work notice is in rectangle shape. The notice was written on ordinary white paper, mimeographed in vertical form and bound together in book form. The content is divided into ten pieces and includes the responsible areas and contact numbers of all the rescue substations. The notice was printed and distributed by the central rescue station of the Health Department of Shanghai Municipal People's Government. It is well preserved and was collected in 1955.

Preserved in Chinese Medical Association/Museum of Chinese Medicine, Shanghai University of Traditional Chinese Medicine

日本住血吸虫病历记录表格

近现代

26 厘米 ×18.3 厘米

长方形，为记录病例表格。该表格是普通白纸红色油印表格，表中详细标明血吸虫的各种检查项目及化验结果栏，该表为空白表格。保存基本完好。1955 年入藏。

中华医学会 / 上海中医药大学医史博物馆藏

Case Record of Schistosoma Japonicum of Japan

Modern Times

26 cm×18.3 cm

This case record is a red mimeographed form on ordinary rectangular white paper, which labels columns of various examination items and laboratory test results of shistosome in details. This is a blank form. It was collected in 1955 and is basically well preserved.

Preserved in Chinese Medical Association/Museum of Chinese Medicine, Shanghai University of Traditional Chinese Medicine

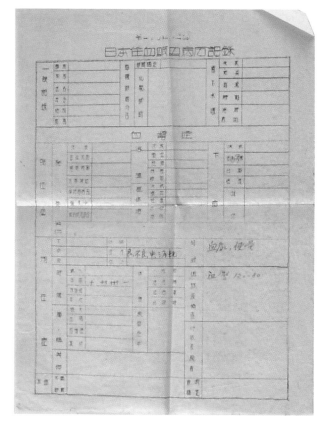

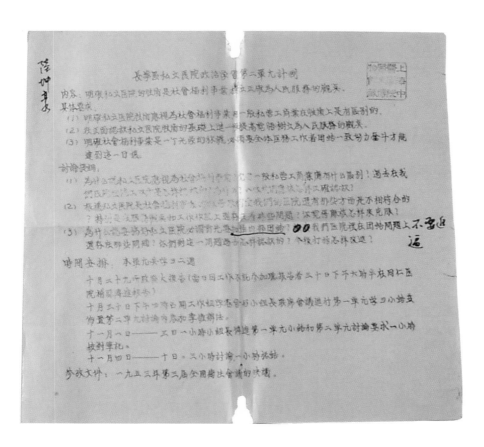

私立医院政治学习计划

近现代

24 厘米 ×22.6 厘米

Study Plan of Politics for Private Hospitals

Modern Times

24 cm×22.6 cm

长方形，为学习计划。普通白纸油印稿，是建国初期上海市长宁区配合当时的资本主义工商业社会主义改造而组织私立医院进行政治学习的一份计划，其中包括学习内容、要求、讨论提纲、时间安排等。该藏左上角有陆坤豪医师的签名。边缘破损。1955 年入藏。

中华医学会 / 上海中医药大学医史博物馆藏

This study plan was written and mimeographed in ordinary rectangular white paper. The study plan of politics for private hospitals was made by Changning District of Shanghai to support the "socialist transformation of capitalist industry and commerce" activity in early years of People's Republic of China. It includes learning contents, requirements, discussion outline, and time arrangement. There is a signature of physician Lu Kunhao on the top left corner of the collection. The margin has been worn out. It was collected in 1955. Preserved in Chinese Medical Association/ Museum of Chinese Medicine, Shanghai University of Traditional Chinese Medicine

各医院区别地址一览表

近现代

42.4 厘米 ×29 厘米

长方形，为职责划分表。普通白纸复写的表格，表中注明上海市各分区救护时救护车负责医院名单及地址，共6个分区29家医院。保存基本完好。1955 年入藏。

中华医学会 / 上海中医药大学医史博物馆藏

List of District Hospitals' Addresses

Modern Times

42.4 cm×29 cm

This table of duty arrangement is made in carbon copy on ordinary rectangular white paper, which contains names and addresses of each hospital responsible for rescue ambulance in all districts of Shanghai. There were 29 hospitals in 6 districts in total. It was collected in 1955 and is basically well preserved.

Preserved in Chinese Medical Association/Museum of Chinese Medicine, Shanghai University of Traditional Chinese Medicine

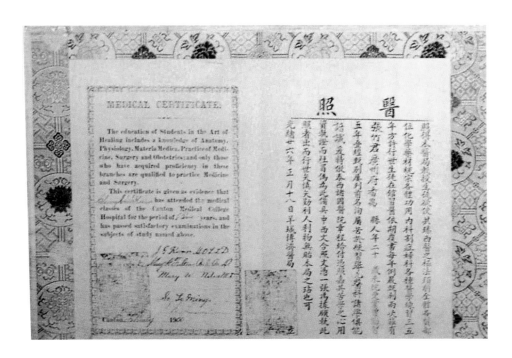

张竹君行医执照

近现代

长 27.5 厘米，宽 21 厘米

光绪二十六年（1900）羊城（广州）博济医局
颁发给张竹君的行医执照。

上海中医药博物馆藏

Medical License of Zhang Zhujun

Modern Times

Length 27.5 cm/ Width 21 cm

This medical license of Zhang Zhujun was issued
by Guangzhou Boji Yiju (a medical bureau) in the
26nd year (1900) of the reign of Emperor Guang Xu.

Preserved in Shanghai Museum of Traditional
Chinese Medicine

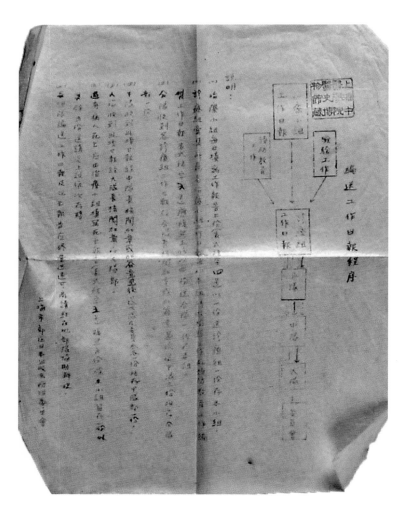

血防工作文件

近现代

27.4 厘米 ×21.3 厘米

Working Document for Schistosomiasis Prevention

Modern Times

27.4 cm×21.3 cm

长方形，为工作规程。该藏为普通白纸油印稿，是中华人民共和国建立初期血吸虫肆虐时上海市郊区日本住血吸虫防治委员会编制的工作日报程序文件。其中包括日报工作程序流程图和说明，反映了当时血防工作的有关情况。边缘有褶皱。1955 年入藏。

中华医学会 / 上海中医药大学医史博物馆藏

This working regulation was mimeographed in ordinary rectangular white paper. It was a procedure file of daily work report made by Shanghai Suburb Committee of Schistosoma Japonicum Prevention during the rampant period of schistosome in early years of PRC. It contains flow charts of daily work procedures and explanations, which reflect the related situations of the schistosome prevention work at that time. The margin is wrinkled and it was collected in 1955.

Preserved in Chinese Medical Association/ Museum of Chinese Medicine, Shanghai University of Traditional Chinese Medicine

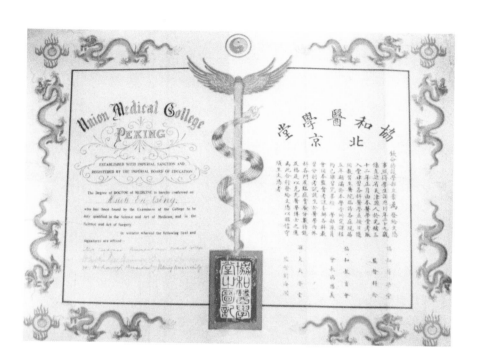

北京协和医学堂毕业证书

近现代

67 厘米 ×51.5 厘米

该藏为 1911 年北京协和医学院发给谢恩增之毕业证书。

上海中医药博物馆藏

Diploma of Peking Union Medical College

Modern Times

67 cm×51.5 cm

It was the diploma of Xie Enzeng awarded by Peking Union Medical College in 1911.

Preserved in Shanghai Museum of Traditional Chinese Medicine

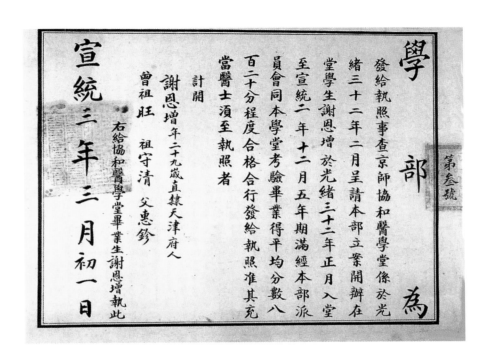

谢恩增医士执照

近现代

长 69 厘米，宽 48 厘米

该藏为宣统三年 (1911) 清政府学部发给北京协和医学堂毕业生谢恩增的医士执照。

上海中医药博物馆藏

Medical License of Xie Enzeng

Modern Times

Length 69 cm/ Width 48 cm

This medical license was issued by the Education Department of the Qing Government to Xie Enzeng, a graduate of Peking Union Medical College, in the third year (1911) of the reign of Emperor Xuan Tong.

Preserved in Shanghai Museum of Traditional Chinese Medicine

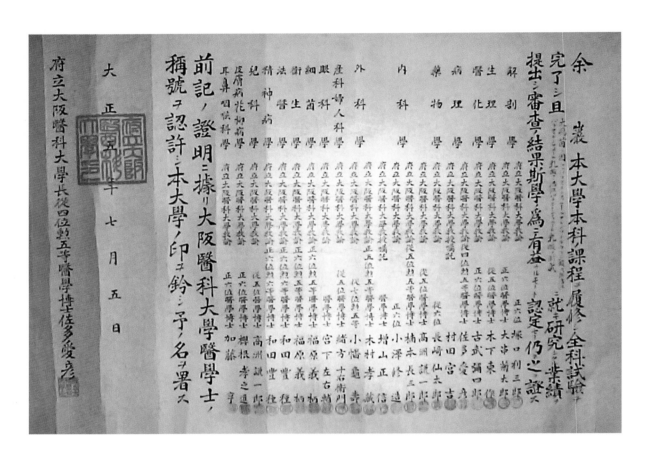

余岩毕业证书

近现代

66.5 厘米 ×51.6 厘米

Diploma of Yu Yan

Modern Times

66.5 cm × 51.6 cm

长方形，为毕业证书。该藏是大阪医科大学于大正五年七月五日颁发给余岩的本科毕业证书。余岩（1879—1954），字云岫，浙江镇海人，近现代医学家。1955 年入藏。保存基本完好。

中华医学会 / 上海中医药大学医史博物馆藏

This rectangular diploma was issued by Osaka Medical College for Yu Yan's Bachelor degree on July 5, the 5th year of Taisho period. Yu Yan (1879–1954), pseudonym Yunxiu, born in Zhenhai, Zhejiang Province, was a medical scientist in modern times. It was collected in 1955 and is basically well preserved.

Preserved in Chinese Medical Association/ Museum of Chinese Medicine, Shanghai University of Traditional Chinese Medicine

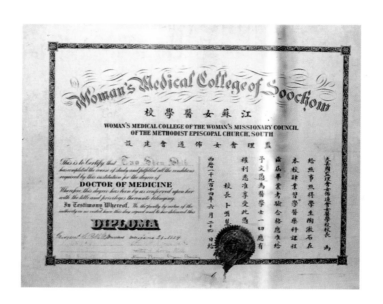

江苏女医学校毕业证书

近现代

长 58 厘米，宽 42 厘米

该证书系美国监理会女布道会设立的江苏女医学校所发医学士文凭。陶漱石捐赠。

上海中医药博物馆藏

Diploma of Women's Medical College of Soochow

Modern Times

Length 58 cm/ Width 42 cm

It was a diploma of Bachelor of Medicine issued by Woman's Medical College of Soochow set up by the Woman's Missionary Council of the Methodist Episcopal Church. It was donated by Tao Shushi.

Preserved in Shanghai Museum of Traditional Chinese Medicine

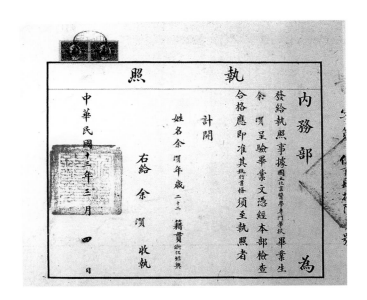

余瀗行医执照

近现代

长 45 厘米，宽 37 厘米

国民政府内务部所发。余瀗捐赠。余瀗（1903— ），浙江绍兴人，民国十三年三月四日，毕业于国立北京中医学专门学校。

上海中医药博物馆藏

Medical License of Yu He

Modern Times

Length 45 cm/ Width 37 cm

The license was issued by the Ministry of Internal Affairs of Republic of China Government. It was donated by Yu He (1903-), Who was born in Shaoxing, Zhejiang Province, and graduated from National Beijing Specialized School of Chinese Medicine on March 4th, the 13th year of the Republic of China (1924).

Preserved in Shanghai Museum of Traditional Chinese Medicine

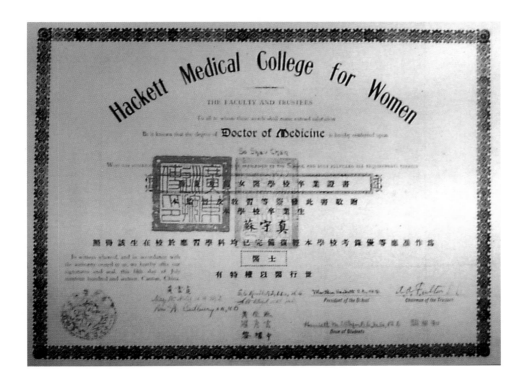

广东夏葛女医学校卒业证书

近现代

64 厘米 ×49.5 厘米

Graduate Certificate of Hackett Medical College for Women

Modern Times

64 cm×49.5 cm

长方形，为证书。该藏为 1916 年学员苏守
真的卒业证书，是由 1901 年美国人夏葛在
广州捐款创建的中国第一所女子医学校——
广东夏葛女医学校给学员颁发的卒业证书，
中英文对照。保存基本完好。1952 年入藏。

中华医学会 / 上海中医药大学医史博物馆藏

This certificate is in rectangular shape. The
collection was the student Su Shouzhen's
graduate certificate issued by Hackett Medical
College for Women, China's first medical
college for women, which was donated and
founded by an American E.A.K. Hackett in
1901. The cerrificate is in both Chinese and
English and basically well preserved. It was
collected in 1952.

Preserved in Chinese Medical Association/
Museum of Chinese Medicine, Shanghai
University of Traditional Chinese Medicine

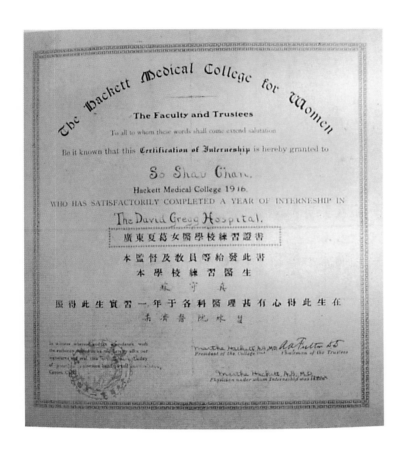

广东夏葛女医学校练习证书

近现代

34.5 厘米 ×32 厘米

Certificate of Internship of Hackett Medical College for Women

Modern Times

34.5 cm×32 cm

长方形，为证书。该藏为 1916 年学员苏守

真的练习（实习）证书，是由 1901 年美国

人夏葛在广州捐款创建的中国第一所女子医

学校——广东夏葛女医学校给学员颁发的练

习证书，中英文对照。保存基本完好。1952 年

入藏。

中华医学会 / 上海中医药大学医史博物馆藏

This certificate is in rectangular shape. This
collection was the student Su Shouzhen's
certificate of internship issued by Hackett
Medical College for Women, China's first
medical college for women, which was donated
and founded by an American E.A.K. Hackett
in 1901. The certificate is in both Chinese and
English and mostly well preserved. It was
collected in 1952.

Preserved in Chinese Medical Association/
Museum of Chinese Medicine, Shanghai
University of Traditional Chinese Medicine

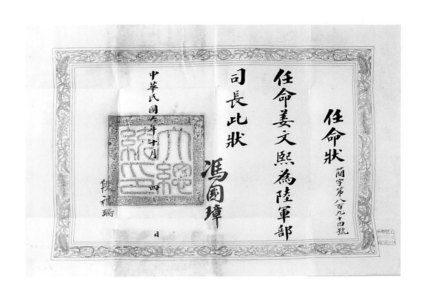

姜文熙任命状

近现代

49 厘米 ×30.2 厘米

长方形，为民国六年十月四日任命姜文熙为陆军部（军医）司长的任命状，钤有大总统印和冯国璋、段祺瑞蓝色名章，标号为"简字第 894 号"。保存基本完好。1956 年入藏。

中华医学会 / 上海中医药大学医史博物馆藏

Jiang Wenxi's Warrant of Appointment

Modern Times

49 cm×30.2 cm

This warrant of appointment is in rectangular shape. This warrant was to appoint Jiang Wenxi as the director of the Department of the (Medical) Army on October 4, the sixth year of the Republic of China. There are also the seal of the president as well as the signature seals of Feng Guozhang and Duan Qirui. Its number is "Jian Zi No. 894". It was collected in 1956 and is basically well preserved.

Preserved in Chinese Medical Association/Museum of Chinese Medicine, Shanghai University of Traditional Chinese Medicine

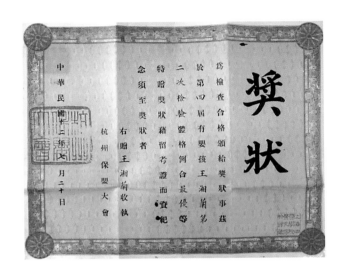

保婴大会奖状

近现代

30.5 厘米 ×26.2 厘米

长方形，为奖状。该藏是中华民国十二年七月二十日第四届杭州保婴大会奖给王湘兰获得最优等体格的奖状，末端有杭州保婴大会落款并钤印。保存完好。1955 年入藏。

中华医学会 / 上海中医药大学医史博物馆藏

Certificate of Merit from Meeting for Baby Protection

Modern

30.5 cm×26.2 cm

This certification of merit is in rectangular shape. This collection was the certificate of "The Best Physique" to Wang Xianglan, awarded by the Fourth Meeting for Baby Protection in Hangzhou on July 20, the 12th year of Republic of China. The Meeting for Baby Protection inscribed and affixed a seal at the end of the certificate. It was collected in 1955 and is well preserved.

Preserved in Chinese Medical Association/Museum of Chinese Medicine, Shanghai University of Traditional Chinese Medicine

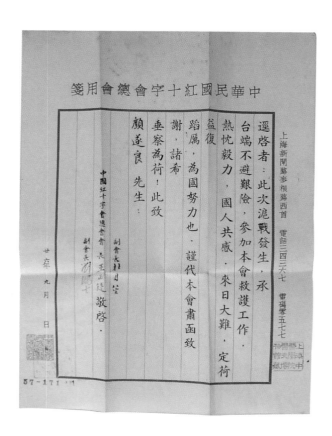

中国红十字会谢函

近现代

28.7 厘米 ×21.8 厘米

Thanks Letter from the Red Cross Society

Modern Times

28.7 cm×21.8 cm

长方形，为谢函。该藏用中华民国红十字会总会用笺印刷填写，是中国红十字会总会于民国二十六年九月给颜遂良的致谢函，以感谢他在沪战发生时参加该会救护工作事宜，末有该会正副会长落款。保存完好。1957 年入藏。

中华医学会 / 上海中医药大学医史博物馆藏

This letter was written and printed on the exclusive rectangular writing paper of Red Cross Society of Republic of China. It was a thanks letter from Red Cross Society of Republic of China to Yan Suiliang in September, the 26th year of Republic of China for his participation in the Society's rescue work during the war in Shanghai. Chairman and Vice-Chairman of the Society were inscribed at the end of the letter. It was collected in 1957 and is still well preserved.

Preserved in Chinese Medical Association/Museum of Chinese Medicine, Shanghai University of Traditional Chinese Medicine

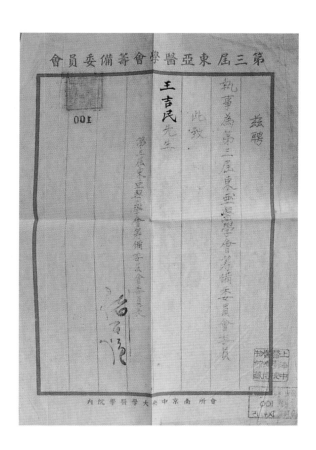

王吉民聘书

近现代

28.2 厘米 ×19.5 厘米

Letter of Appointment for Wang Jimin

Modern Times

28.2 cm×19.5 cm

长方形，为聘书。用"第三届东亚医学会筹备委
员会用笺"油印填写而成，为该委员会聘请王吉
民为委员的聘书，文末有该会委员长落款。保存
完好。1952 年入藏。

中华医学会 / 上海中医药大学医史博物馆藏

Mimeographed and written on the exclusive
rectangular writing paper of the Preparatory
Committee of the Third Eastern Asia Medicine
Meeting, this letter of appointment was to engage
Wang Jimin as a committee member. Chairman
of the committee inscribed his signiture at the end
of the letter. It was collected in 1952 and is well
preserved.

Preserved in Chinese Medical Association/Museum
of Chinese Medicine, Shanghai University of
Traditional Chinese Medicine

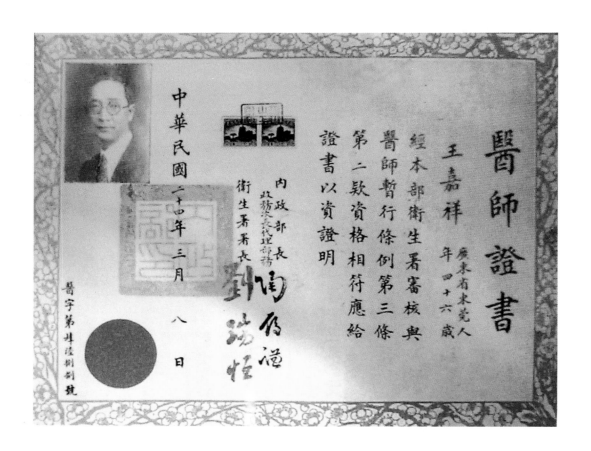

王吉民医师证书

近现代

长 44.3 厘米，宽 36.5 厘米

Physician Certificate of Wang Jimin

Modern Times

Length 44.3 cm/ Width 36.5 cm

长方形，为证书。该藏为国民政府内政部、卫生署颁发给王吉民的医师证书。保存完好。1952 年入藏。

中华医学会 / 上海中医药大学医史博物馆藏

The certificate is in rectangular shape. This collection was the physician certificate for Wang Jimin issued by the Ministry of Internal Affairs and the Department of Health of Republic of China Government. It was collected in 1952 and is well preserved.

Preserved in Chinese Medical Association/ Museum of Chinese Medicine, Shanghai University of Traditional Chinese Medicine

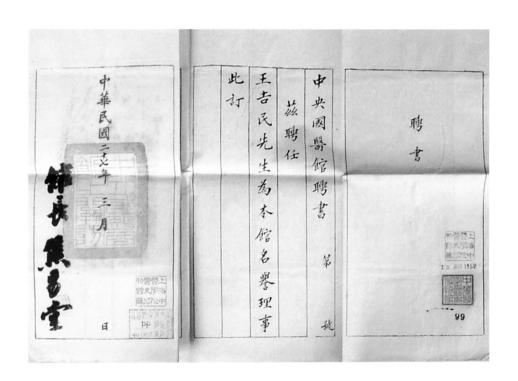

王吉民聘书

近现代

68.2 厘米 ×27.6 厘米

Letter of Appointment for Wang Jimin

Modern Times

68.2 cm×27.6 cm

长方形，为聘书。普通白纸毛笔填写。该藏
是民国二十七年中央国医馆聘请王吉民为该
馆名誉理事聘书。文末有馆长落款和该馆图
记。保存完好。1952 年入藏。

中华医学会 / 上海中医药大学医史博物馆藏

The letter of appointment was written with
brush on ordinary rectangular white pape by the
Central Traditional Chinese Medical Institute
to engage Wang Jimin as an honorary council
member in the 27th year of Republic of China.
The signature of the head and the seal of the
institute were affixed at the end of the letter. It
was collected in 1952 and is well preserved.
Preserved in Chinese Medical Association/
Museum of Chinese Medicine, Shanghai
University of Traditional Chinese Medicine

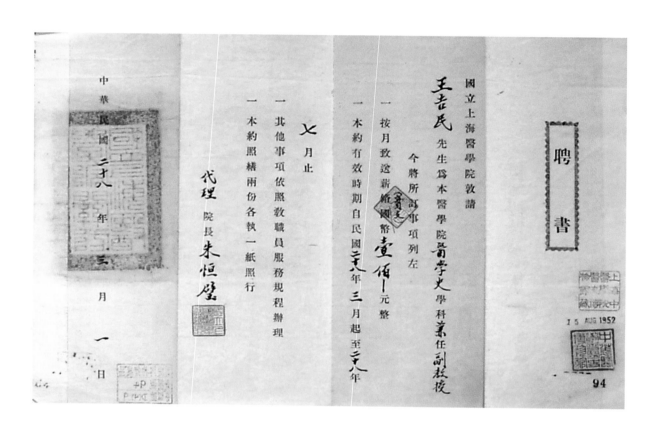

王吉民聘书

近现代

36 厘米 ×21.4 厘米

The Letter of Appointment for Wang Jimin

Modern Times

36 cm×21.4 cm

长方形，为聘书。该聘书是民国二十八年三月一日国立上海医学院聘请王吉民为医学史副教授的聘书。文末有代理院长落款及印章，并钤国立上海医学院关防章。保存完好。1952 年入藏。

中华医学会 / 上海中医药大学医史博物馆藏

The letter of appointment is in rectangle shape. The letter was to appoint Wang Jimin as an associate professor of medical history in Shanghai National Medical College on March 1, the 28th year of Republic of China. The deputy dean inscribed the name and affixed a seal at the end of the letter. There is also the official seal of Shanghai National Medical College at the end of the letter. It was collected in 1952 and is well preserved.

Preserved in Chinese Medical Association/ Museum of Chinese Medicine, Shanghai University of Traditional Chinese Medicine

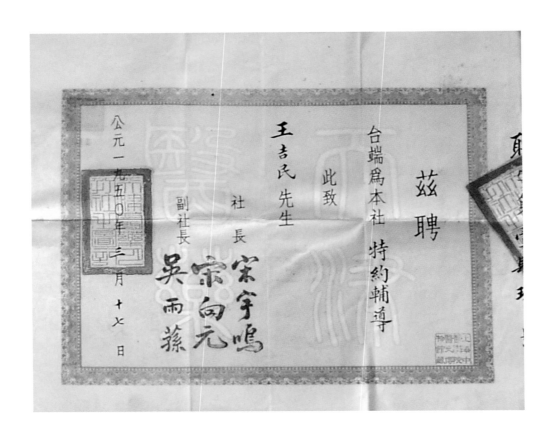

王吉民聘书

近现代

31.7 厘米 ×27 厘米

Letter of Appointment of Wang Jimin

Modern Times

31.7 cm×27 cm

长方形，为聘书。该藏为 1950 年 3 月 17 日《天津医药月刊》社聘请王吉民先生为该社特约辅导的聘书。文末有社长、副社长落款和该社图记。王吉民（1889—1972），广东东莞人，1910 年毕业于香港西医大学堂，曾与伍连德合著《中国医学史》，后被推选为医史委员会主席和中华医史学会会长，1938 年创办中国第一家医史博物馆，并任馆长。保存完好。1952 年入藏。

中华医学会 / 上海中医药大学医史博物馆藏

The rectangular paper is a letter of appointment, showing that in March 17, 1950, *Tianjin Medical Monthly* Editorial office employed Wang Jimin as the Speical Tutor for their office. There are signatures of the president and vice-president and stamp of the magazine on it. Wang Jimin (1889-1972) was born in Dongguan City, Guangdong Province, and graduated in 1910 from Hongkong Western Medical School. He co-authored *China Medical History* with Wu Lien-Teh. He was elected as the Chairman of the Medical History Committee and the President of Chinese Medical History Association. In 1938, he established the first Museum of Chinese Medicine in China, and served as the president. The paper is preserved well. It was collected in 1952.

Preserved in Chinese Medical Association/Museum of Chinese Medicine, Shanghai University of Traditional Chinese Medicine

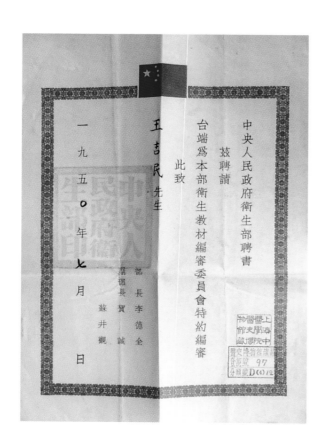

王吉民聘书

近现代

27.2 厘米 ×19.8 厘米

Letter of Appointment of Wang Jimin

Modern Times

27.2 cm×19.8 cm

长方形，为聘书。该聘书是 1950 年 7 月中央
人民政府卫生部聘请王吉民为卫生教材编审委
员会特约编审的聘书。文末有卫生部部长、副
部长落款及中央人民政府卫生部印章。保存完
好。1952 年入藏。

中华医学会 / 上海中医药大学医史博物馆藏

The rectangular paper is a letter of appointment,
showing that in July, 1950, Central Government
Ministry of Health employed Wang Jimin as
the Special editor for Medical Textbook Editing
Committee. There are signatures of the minister
and vice-minister and stamp of the ministry on
it. The paper is preserved well. It was collected
in 1952.

Preserved in Chinese Medical Association/
Museum of Chinese Medicine, Shanghai
University of Traditional Chinese Medicine

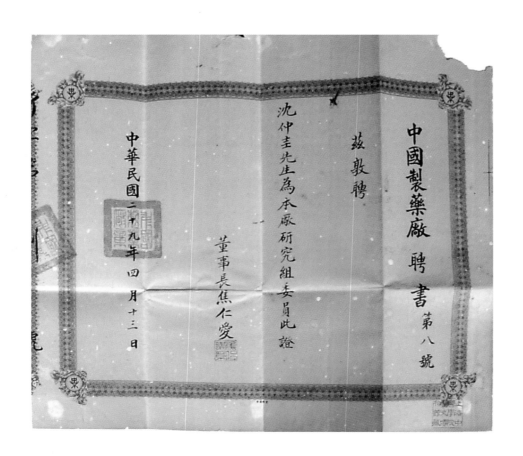

沈仲圭聘书

近现代

33.6 厘米 ×30.1 厘米

Letter of Appointment of Shen Zhonggui

Modern Times

33.6 cm×30.1 cm

长方形，为聘书。该聘书是民国二十九年四月十三日中国制药厂聘请沈仲圭为该厂研究组委员的证书。文末有该厂董事长落款及印章，并钤中国制药厂章。沈仲圭（1901—　　），浙江杭州人，早年从王香岩学医，曾任教于上海国医学院，解放后曾在中医研究院工作，主要著作有《养生琐谈》《仲圭医论汇选》《中国小儿传染病学》等。已破损。1952 年入藏。

中华医学会 / 上海中医药大学医史博物馆藏

This rectangular letter of appointment shows that on April 13 of the 29th year of the Republic of China, Chinese Pharmaceutical Manufacturer employed Shen Zhonggui as a member of its research group. There are chairman's signature and manufacturer's stamp on it. Shen Zhonggui was born in 1901 in Hangzhou City, Zhejiang Province. When he was young, he was taught medicine by Wang Xiangyan. He once was employed as a teacher in Shanghai College of Traditional Chinese Medicine. After 1949, he worked at the Institute of Traditional Chinese Medicine. His major works include *Yang Sheng Suo Tan* (On Keeping Health), *Zhong Gui Yi Lun Hui Suan* (Collection of Shen Zhanggui's Medical Essays), and *Pediatric Infectious Diseases in China*, etc. It was collected in 1952. The collection has been worn out.

Preserved in Chinese Medical Association/Museum of Chinese Medicine, Shanghai University of Traditional Chinese Medicine

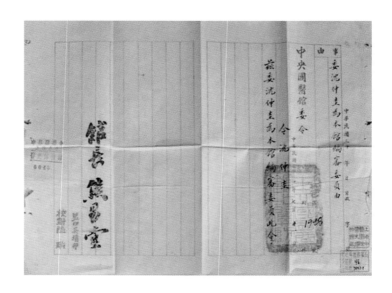

委沈仲圭令

近现代

37.4 厘米 ×26.2 厘米

长方形，为聘书，是民国 31 年 7 月 21 日中央国医馆委任沈仲圭为该馆编审委员会委员令。文末有馆长焦易堂落款，并钤中央国医馆关防。保存完好。1952 年入藏。

中华医学会 / 上海中医药大学医史博物馆藏

Letter of Appointment of Shen Zhonggui

Modern Times

37.4 cm×26.2 cm

This rectangular letter of appointment shows that on July 21 of the 31st year of the Republic of China, the Central Traditional Chinese Medical Institute appointed Shen Zhonggui as a member of its Editorial Review Board. There are the signature of President Jiao Yitang and the institute's stamp. It is preserved well. It was collected in 1952.

Preserved in Chinese Medical Association/Museum of Chinese Medicine, Shanghai University of Traditional Chinese Medicine

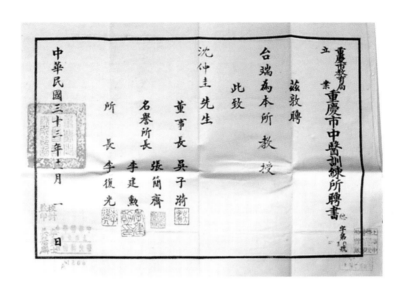

沈仲圭聘书

近现代

34.6 厘米 × 25 厘米

纸张形，为聘书，是民国三十三年十一月一日重庆市中医训练所聘请沈仲圭为教授的聘书。文末有该所董事长、名誉所长、所长落款和印章，并有重庆市中医训练所钤记。保存完好。1952 年入藏。

中华医学会 / 上海中医药大学医史博物馆藏

Letter of Appointment of Shen Zhonggui

Modern Times

34.6 cm × 25 cm

This letter of appointment shows that on November 1 of the 33rd year of the Republic of China, Chongqing Chinese Medical Training School appointed Shen Zhonggui as the professor. There are signatures of the President, the Honorary Director and the Director, and the stamp of the school. It is preserved well. It was collected in 1952.

Preserved in Chinese Medical Association/Museum of Chinese Medicine, Shanghai University of Traditional Chinese Medicine

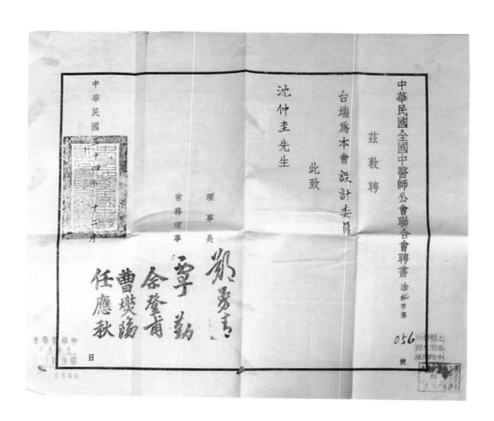

沈仲圭聘书

近现代

34.6 厘米 ×28.3 厘米

Letter of Appointment of Shen Zhonggui

Modern Times

34.6 cm×28.3 cm

纸张形，为聘书，是民国三十四年十二月全国中医师公会联合会聘请沈仲圭为设计委员的聘书。文末有该会理事长、常务理事落款，并钤中华民国全国中医师公会联合会图记。保存完好。1952 年入藏。

中华医学会 / 上海中医药大学医史博物馆藏

This letter of appointment shows that in December of the 34th year of the Pepublic of China, National Association of Traditional Chinese Medicine Doctors' Union appointed Shen Zhonggui as a member of the Design Committee. There are the signatures of the President and the Managing Director, and the stamp of the union. It was collected in 1952 and is preserved well.

Preserved in Chinese Medical Association/ Museum of Chinese Medicine, Shanghai University of Traditional Chinese Medicine

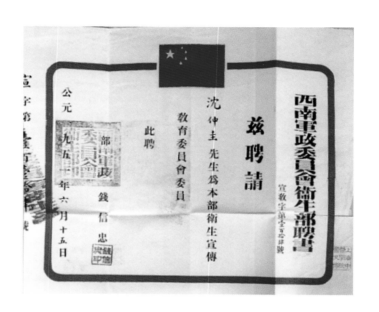

沈仲圭聘书

近现代

30 厘米 ×25 厘米

长方形，为聘书。该藏是 1951 年 6 月 15 日西南军政委员会卫生部聘请沈仲圭为卫生宣传教育委员会委员的聘书，文末有校长落款及印章，并钤西南军政委员会印。保存完好。1952 年入藏。

中华医学会 / 上海中医药大学医史博物馆藏

Letter of Appointment of Shen Zhonggui

Modern Times

30 cm×25 cm

This letter of appointment shows that on June 15, 1951, Health Department of the Southwest Military Administrative Committee appointed Shen Zhonggui as a member of the Health Propaganda and Education Committee. There are the signature of the President and the seal of the Southwest Military Administrative Committee. It was collected in 1952 and is preserved well.

Preserved in Chinese Medical Association/Museum of Chinese Medicine, Shanghai University of Traditional Chinese Medicine

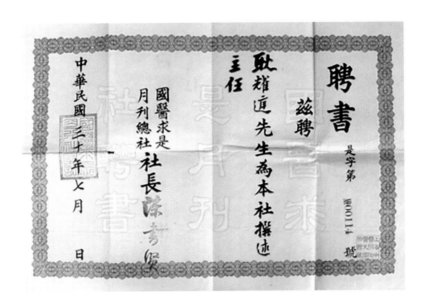

耿耀庭聘书

近现代

39 厘米 ×26.8 厘米

长方形，为聘书，用普通白纸套色印刷填写而成，是民国 30 年 7 月《国医求是月刊》总社聘请耿耀庭为该社撰述主任的聘书。文末有社长落款和该社图记。保存完好。1955 年入藏。

中华医学会 / 上海中医药大学医史博物馆藏

Letter of Appointment of Geng Yaoting

Modern Times

39 cm×26.8 cm

This letter of appointment is in a normal rectangular white paper in polychrome printing, showing that in July 1941, the editorial headquarter of *Guo Yi Qiu Shi Yue Kan* (a Chinese medicine monthly journal) appointed Geng Yaoting as the Writing Director. In the end, there are the signature of the Director and the stamp of the journal. It was collected in 1955 and is preserved well.

Preserved in Chinese Medical Association/Museum of Chinese Medicine, Shanghai University of Traditional Chinese Medicine

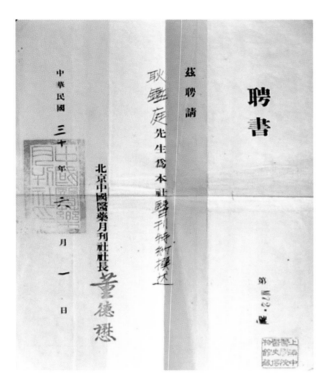

耿鉴庭聘书

近现代

26.6 厘米 ×19.1 厘米

长方形，为聘书。该聘书用普通白纸铅印填写而成。是民国三十年六月一日《中国医药月刊》社聘请耿鉴庭为该社医刊特约撰述的聘书。文末有社长落款及该社红色图章。保存完好。1955 年入藏。

中华医学会 / 上海中医药大学医史博物馆藏

Letter of Appointment of Geng Jianting

Modern Times

26.6 cm×19.1 cm

This letter of appointment is in a normal rectangular white paper and in lead print, showing that on June 1, the 30th year of the Republic of China 1941, the editorial office of *Chinese Medicine Monthly* appointed Geng Jianting as a special writer of the Medical Column. In the end, there are the signature of the Director and the red stamp of the journal. It was collected in 1955 and is preserved well.

Preserved in Chinese Medical Association/Museum of Chinese Medicine, Shanghai University of Traditional Chinese Medicine

耿监庭医师聘书

近现代

27.5 厘米 ×17.4 厘米

长方形，为聘书。该藏用江都县中医师公会用笺油印填写，为民国三十五年二月聘任耿鉴庭医师为江都县中医师公会处方鉴定委员会委员的聘书，文末有该公会款识。保存完好。1955 年入藏。

　　中华医学会 / 上海中医药大学医史博物馆藏

Letter of Appointment of Physician Geng Jianting

Modern Times

27.5 cm×17.4 cm

This rectangular mineographed letter shows that it was authorized in February 1946 by Jiangdu Traditional Chinese Medicine Doctor Union to appoint Geng Jianting as a member of its Prescription Examination Committee. In the end, there is the union's stamp. It was collected in 1955 and is preserved well.

Preserved in Chinese Medical Association/Museum of Chinese Medicine, Shanghai University of Traditional Chinese Medicine

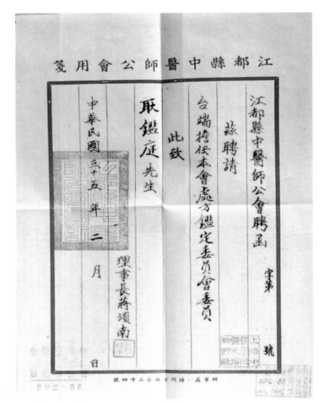

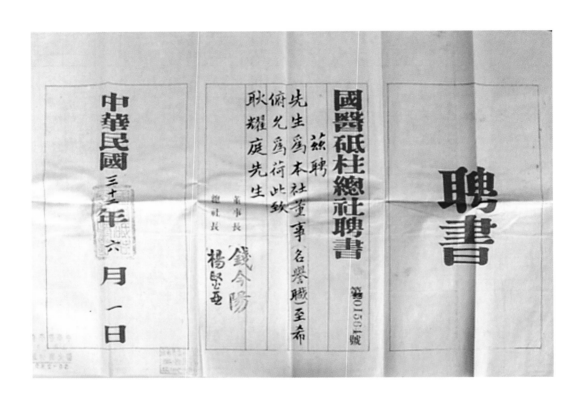

耿耀庭聘书

近现代

44 厘米 ×29 厘米

Letter of Appointment of Geng Yaoting

Modern Times

44 cm×29 cm

长方形，为聘书。该藏用普通白纸印刷填写，为《国医砥柱》总社聘任耿耀庭为该社董事的聘书。文末有该社董事长、总社长落款及图记款识。保存完好。1955 年入藏。

中华医学会 / 上海中医药大学医史博物馆藏

This letter of appointment in a normal rectangular white paper shows that *Pillar Chinese Medicine Monthly* the editorial headquarter of appointed Geng Yaoting as the Director. In the end, there are signatures of the journal's board director and general director as well as the stamp of the journal. It was collected in 1955 and is preserved well.

Preserved in Chinese Medical Association/ Museum of Chinese Medicine, Shanghai University of Traditional Chinese Medicine

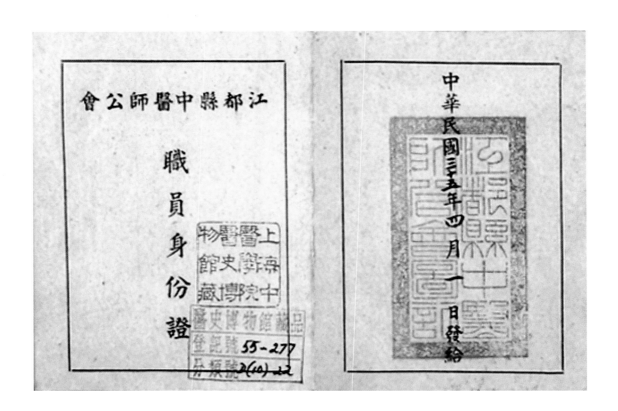

江都县耿鉴庭中医师公会职员身份证

近现代

15 厘米 ×9.5 厘米

Identification Card of Geng Jianting as the Member of Jiangdu TCM Doctor Union

Modern Times

15 cm×9.5 cm

长方形，为证件。白色对折，封面印有"江都县中医师公会职员身份证"字样；背面印"中华民国三十五年四月一日发给"并钤"江都县中医师公会图记"章。证内面填有持证人姓名、性别、年龄、籍贯、住址、职别，且粘照片钤印章。该藏是发给江都县医师耿鉴庭的证件。保存完好。1955 年入藏。

中华医学会 / 上海中医药大学医史博物馆藏

The cover of this white and folio piece of paper shows it is an identity card of the Member of Jiangdu TCM Doctor Union. On the back it is printed with characters showing that it was authorized on April 1 of the 35th year of the Republic of China and with the seal of Jiangdu TCM Doctor Union. There can be seen the cardholder's name, gender, age, place of origin, address, job title, his photo and his seal. The card was issued to Jiangdu Physician Geng Jianting. It was collected in 1955 and is preserved well.

Preserved in Chinese Medical Association/ Museum of Chinese Medicine, Shanghai University of Traditional Chinese Medicine

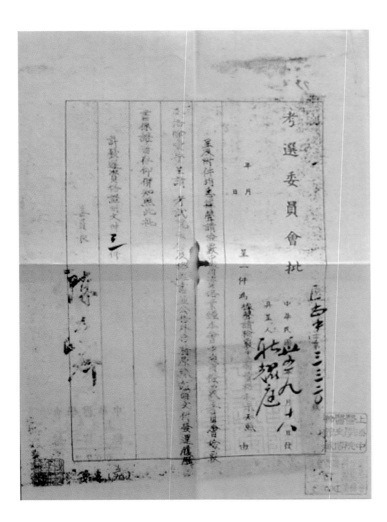

考选委员会批

近现代

26.6 厘米 ×17.6 厘米

Approval Document of Selection Committee

Modern Times

26.6 cm×17.6 cm

长方形，为批文，是中华民国三十五年九月十六日检核耿鉴庭中医师资格及格的批示知照，该证照呈请考试院向耿鉴庭颁发及格证书，并钤公章。保存基本完好。1955 年入藏。

中华医学会 / 上海中医药大学医史博物馆藏

This rectangular document was to officially notify that on September 16 the 35th year of the Republic of China (1946), Geng Jianting had passed the Traditional Chinese Medicine Physician Qualification Examination, and it was to inform that the examination council should issue the certificate to him. And there is a stamp on it. It was collected in 1955 and is preserved well.
Preserved in Chinese Medical Association/ Museum of Chinese Medicine, Shanghai University of Traditional Chinese Medicine

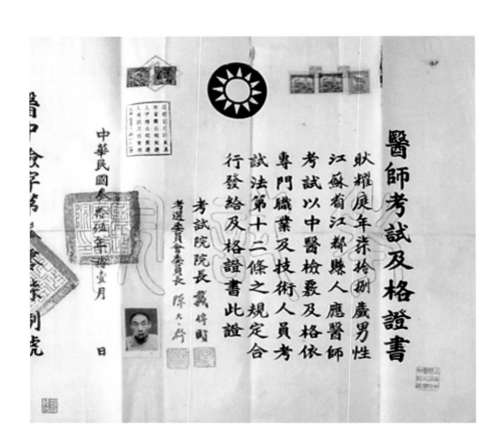

耿鉴庭医师考试及格证书

近现代

42.3 厘米 ×39.4 厘米

Physician Examination Certificate of Geng Jianting

Modern Times

42.3 cm×39.4 cm

长方形，为合格证书，是民国三十五年十一月国民政府考试院颁发给耿鉴庭中医师的考试及格证书。证书上方印有国民党党徽，并粘印花税票五张，面值共计 50 元，下端粘耿鉴庭照片，并钤钢印和国民政府考试院院长和考选委员会委员长的落款与钤记，末尾和骑缝钤国民政府考试院公章。保存基本完好。1952 年入藏。

中华医学会 / 上海中医药大学医史博物馆藏

The rectangular paper is a certificate issued by the Examination Council of the National Government to TCM Physician Geng Jianting in November of the 35th year of the Republic of China. On the upper part there was printed the emblem of Kuo Min Tang, with five revenue stamps pasted on it, worth 50 yuan in total value. On the lower part, Geng's photo was pasted, with embossment and the signatures of the President of the Examination Council of the Republic of China and of the Chairman of Selection Committee and their stamps. The stamp of the Examination Council of the Republic of China can be seen on the perforation. It was collected in 1952 and is basically preserved well.
Preserved in Chinese Medical Association/Museum of Chinese Medicine, Shanghai University of Traditional Chinese Medicine

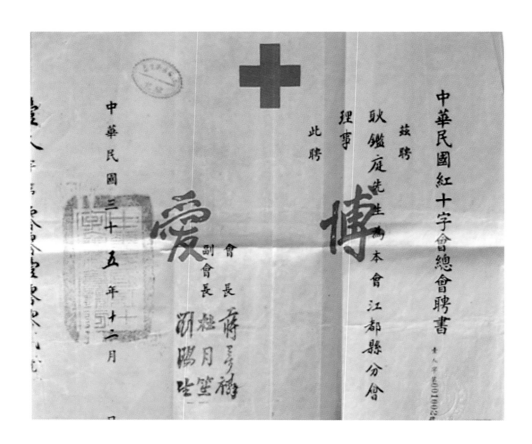

耿鉴庭聘书

近现代

31 厘米 ×26.6 厘米

Letter of Appointment of Geng Jianting

Modern Times

31cm×26.6 cm

纸张形，为聘书。该馆收藏的纸质文献之一，腊光纸印刷填写而成，为民国三十五年十二月中华民国红十字总会聘请耿鉴庭为该会江都县分会理事的聘书，上端印有红十字图案和"博爱"红字，文末有会长、副会长落款并钤中华民国红十字会总会图记，并有该会钢印。保存完好。1955 年入藏。

中华医学会 / 上海中医药大学医史博物馆藏

This letter of appointment printed on double seal paper shows that in December of the 35th year of the Republic of China, the Red Cross of the Republic of China appointed Geng Jianting as a Director of its Jiangdu Branch. On the upper part there are designs of the Red Cross and the red characters "Bo Ai" meaning "fraternity". In the end there are the signatures of the Chairman and the Vice Chairman as well as the stamp and the steel seal of the Red Cross. It was collected in 1955 and is preserved well. Preserved in Chinese Medical Association/ Museum of Chinese Medicine, Shanghai University of Traditional Chinese Medicine

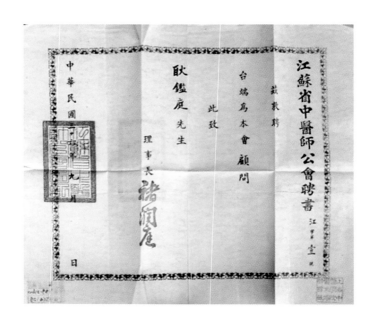

耿鉴庭医师聘书

近现代

29.2 厘米 ×25.4 厘米

长方形，为聘书。该藏用普白纸印刷填写，是江苏省中医师公会聘请耿鉴庭先生为该会顾问的聘书，文末有该会图记和理事长签章。保存完好。1959 年入藏。

中华医学会 / 上海中医药大学医史博物馆藏

Letter of Appointment of Physician Geng Jianting

Modern Times

29.2 cm×25.4 cm

This letter of appointment in rectangular white paper shows that Jiangsu TCM Physician Union appointed Geng Jianting as a counselor. In the end there are the signature of the Chairman and the union's stamp. It was collected in 1959 and is preserved well.

Preserved in Chinese Medical Association/Museum of Chinese Medicine, Shanghai University of Traditional Chinese Medicine

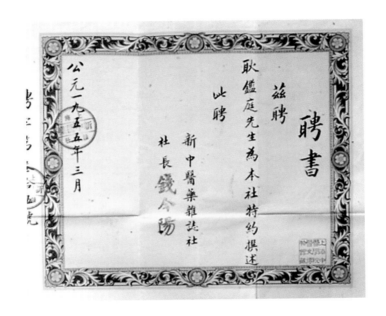

耿鉴庭聘书

近现代

29.2 厘米 ×26.1 厘米

长方形，为聘书。该藏用普通白纸套色印刷填写，为 1955 年 3 月《上海新中医药杂志》社聘请耿鉴庭先生为特约撰述的聘书。文末有该社及社长落款，并钤该社蓝色图章。保存完好。1955 年入藏。

中华医学会 / 上海中医药大学医史博物馆藏

Letter of Appointment of Geng Jianting

Modern Times

29.2 cm×26.1 cm

This letter of appointment in normal rectangular white paper with polychrome printing shows that in March 1955, the editorial office of *Shanghai New TCM Magazine* appointed Geng Jianting as a special writer. In the end there are the signature of the Director and the magazine office with the blue seal. It was collected in 1955 and is preserved well. Preserved in Chinese Medical Association/Museum of Chinese Medicine, Shanghai University of Traditional Chinese Medicine

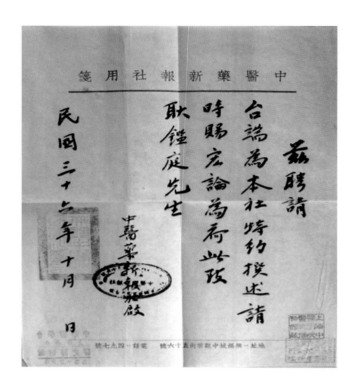

耿鉴庭医师聘书

近现代

29.2 厘米 ×20.2 厘米

长方形，为聘书。该藏用《中医药新报》社用笺写就，为聘任耿鉴庭医师为该社特邀撰述的聘书，文末有该社款识。保存完好。1955 年入藏。

　中华医学会 / 上海中医药大学医史博物馆藏

Letter of Appointment of Physician Geng Jianting

Modern Times

29.2 cm×20.2 cm

This letter of appointment was authorized by "*Zhong Yi Yao Xin Bao She*" (a newspaper office) to appoint Geng Jianting as a special writer. In the end there is inscriptions of the newspaper. It was collected in 1955 and is preserved well.

Preserved in Chinese Medical Association/ Museum of Chinese Medicine, Shanghai University of Traditional Chinese Medicine

耿鉴庭医师聘书

近现代

28 厘米 ×17.3 厘米

长方形，为聘书。该藏用苏北中等学校教师暑期研究会用笺写就，是聘任耿鉴庭医师为该会医疗室主任的聘书，文末有该会款识。1959 年入藏。保存完好。

中华医学会 / 上海中医药大学医史博物馆藏

Letter of Appointment of Physician Geng Jianting

Modern Times

28 cm×17.3 cm

This letter of appointment was authorized by Summer Institute of Teachers of Northern Jiangsu Secondary School to appoint Geng Jianting as the director of its medical office. In the end there is the school's inscription. It was collected in 1959 and is preserved well.

Preserved in Chinese Medical Association/Museum of Chinese Medicine, Shanghai University of Traditional Chinese Medicine

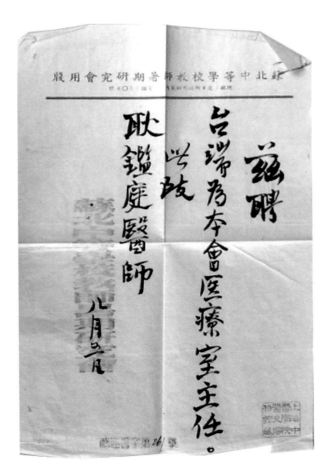

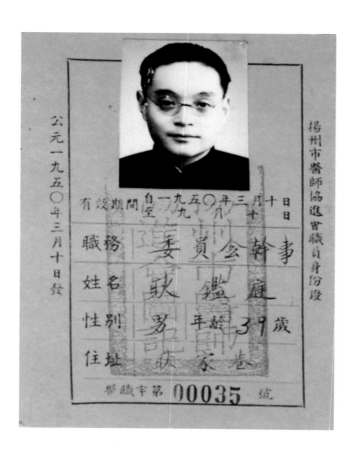

扬州市医师协进会职员身份证

近现代

10.3 厘米 ×7.6 厘米

Identification Card for the Member of Yangzhou Physician Council

Modern Times

10.3 cm×7.6 cm

卡片式，为证件。该藏用粉红色普通卡片铅印
而成，一面印有"扬州市医师协进会职员身份
证"字样和红十字图案；另面粘耿鉴庭照片，
照片钤"扬州市医师协进会图记"骑缝章，并
填有持证人姓名、性别、年龄、住址、职务
和有效期等栏目。保存完好。1955 年入藏。

中华医学会/上海中医药大学医史博物馆藏

The pink paper with lead print is an identification
card. On one side there are characters showing
that it is an Identification Card of the Member
of Yangzhou Physician Council, with design of
the Red Cross. On the other side, the photo of its
holder was pasted with the stamp of Yangzhou
Physician Council on the perforation. It shows
the holder's name, gender, age, address, job title
and the validity date. It was collected in 1955 and
is preserved well.

Preserved in Chinese Medical Association/
Museum of Chinese Medicine, Shanghai
University of Traditional Chinese Medicine

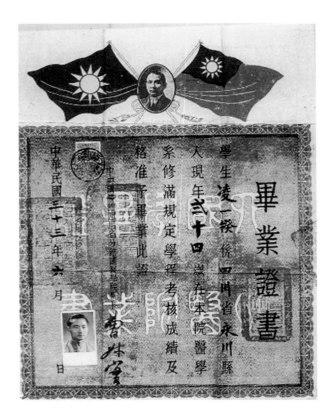

四川国医学院毕业证书

近现代

46 厘米 ×34.5 厘米

四川国医学院创建于 1936 年。此为该院第十一期学生凌一揆毕业证书。

成都中医药大学中医药传统文化博物馆藏

The diploma of Sichuan College of Traditional Chinese Medicine

Modern Times

46 cm×34.5 cm

Sichuan College of Traditional Chinese Medicine was established in 1936. This diploma is issued to Ling Yikui, one of the eleventh batch of its graduates.

Preserved in Chinese Medical Association/Museum of Chinese Medicine, Shanghai University of Traditional Chinese Medicine

致庞京周贺年片

近现代

18 厘米 ×9.1 厘米

卡片形，为贺年卡。粉红色边框贺年卡，是 1947 年临大二乙分发同济大学全体学生给庞京周先生的贺年卡，表达了学生们对庞京周先生帮助他们分业至同济大学一事的感谢之情和新年祝贺。另有庞京周亲笔附件。保存完好。1952 年入藏。

中华医学会 / 上海中医药大学医史博物馆藏

New Year Card to Pang Jingzhou

Modern Times

18 cm×9.1 cm

This New Year card with pink frame was sent to Pang Jingzhou by his second-year students in Tongji University, showing their gratitude for his help in their admittance to Tongji University as well as their New Year's greetings. It is also attached with Pang Jingzhou's hand-written accessory. It was collected in 1952 and is preserved well.

Preserved in Chinese Medical Association/Museum of Chinese Medicine, Shanghai University of Traditional Chinese Medicine

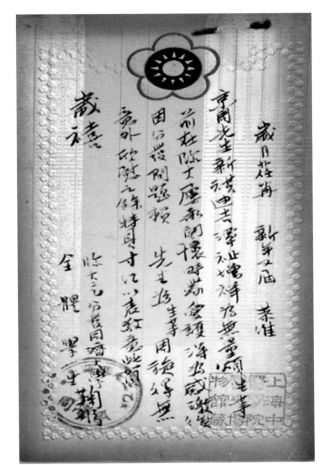

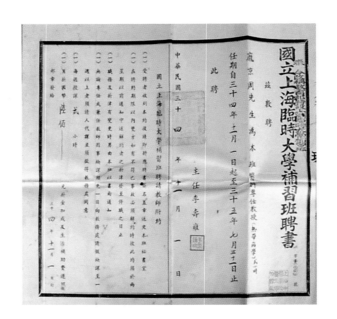

庞京周聘书

近现代

34 厘米 × 30.6 厘米

长方形，为聘书，是民国三十四年十一月一日国立上海临时大学补习班聘请庞京周为分班主任的聘书。聘词后有主任落款印章和教育部特设上海临时大学补习班钤记。后有教师附约。保存完好。1952 年入藏。

中华医学会 / 上海中医药大学医史博物馆藏

Letter of Appointment of Pang Jingzhou

Modern Times

34 cm×30.6 cm

This rectangular letter of appointment shows that in November 1945, National Shanghai Temporary College Training Class appointed Pang Jingzhou as the teacher in charge. Following the employment statement there are the inscriptions and seals of the Director and the class. There is accessory contract attached. It was collected in 1952 and is preserved well.

Preserved in Chinese Medical Association/Museum of Chinese Medicine, Shanghai University of Traditional Chinese Medicine

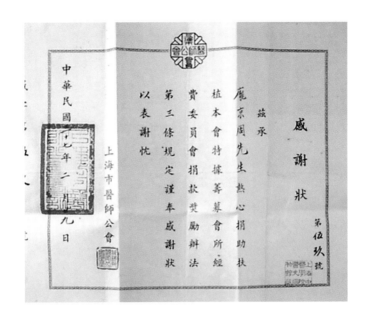

上海市医师公会致庞京周感谢状

近现代

27.6 厘米 ×25.5 厘米

长方形，为感谢状。该藏是民国三十七年二月二十九日上海市医师公会颁发给庞京周的感谢状，以谢忱庞先生对该会的热心捐助。文末钤上海市医师公会图章和图记各一枚。保存基本完好。1955 年入藏。

中华医学会 / 上海中医药大学医史博物馆藏

Letter of Thanks to Pang Jingzhou From Shanghai Physician Union

Modern Times

27.6 cm×25.5 cm

This letter of appreciation was issued in February 29 of the 37th year of the Republic of China, by Shanghai Physician Union to Pang Jingzhou, to thank him for his warmhearted donation to Shanghai Physician Union. In the end there are a seal and a stamp of Shanghai Physician Union. It was collected in 1955 and is preserved well.

Preserved in Chinese Medical Association/Museum of Chinese Medicine, Shanghai University of Traditional Chinese Medicine

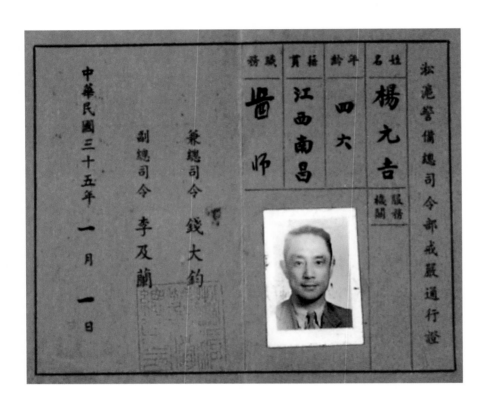

戒严通行证

近现代

13 厘米 ×9.9 厘米

Curfew Pass

Modern Times

13 cm×9.9 cm

证件形，为通行证。粉红色对开，封面印有"淞沪警备总司令部戒严通行证交字第39162"字样。证内一面填有持证人姓名、年龄、籍贯、职务，且粘照片钤钢印；另面印有"中华民国三十五年一月一日兼总司令钱大钧、副总司令李及阑"字样，并钤"淞沪警备总司令"章。该藏是发给江西南昌杨元吉医师的证件。保存完好。1958年入藏。

中华医学会／上海中医药大学医史博物馆藏

The pink and folio paper is a curfew pass. On its cover there are characters meaning that it is a curfew pass authorized by Songhu Garrison Headquarter with "Jiao Zi No. 39162". On the one inner side were written the holder's name, age, place of origin, job title, with his photo pasted and a steal seal. On the other inner side there are characters showing the date January 1 of the 35th year of the Republic of China and the name Qian Dajun, the Commander in Chief, and the name Li Jilan, Deputy Commander in Chief, as well as the seal of "Commander in Chief of Jianghu Garrison Headquarter". It was offered to Physician Yang Yuanji in Nan Chang City, Jiangxi Province. It was collected in 1958 and is preserved well. Preserved in Chinese Medical Association/Museum of Chinese Medicine, Shanghai University of Traditional Chinese Medicine

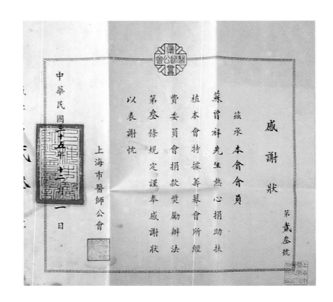

上海市医师公会致苏曾祥感谢状

近现代

27.8 厘米 ×25.7 厘米

长方形，为感谢状。该藏是民国三十五年十二月一日上海市医师公会颁发给苏曾祥的感谢状，以谢忱苏先生对该会的热心捐助，文末钤上海市医师公会图章和图记各一枚。保存基本完好。1955 年入藏。

中华医学会 / 上海中医药大学医史博物馆藏

Letter of Thanks to Su Cengxiang From Shanghai Physician Union

Modern Times

27.8 cm×25.7 cm

This rectangular letter of appreciation was issued on December 1 of the 35th year of the Repubic of China, by Shanghai Physician Union to Su Cengxiang, to thank him for his warmhearted donation to Shanghai Physician Union. In the end there are a seal and a stamp of Shanghai Physician Union. It was collected in 1955 and is preserved well.

Preserved in Chinese Medical Association/Museum of Chinese Medicine, Shanghai University of Traditional Chinese Medicine

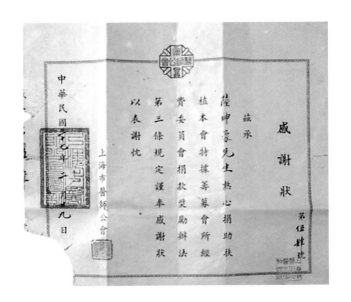

上海市医师公会致陆坤豪感谢状

近现代

27.6 厘米 ×25.5 厘米

长方形，为感谢状。该藏是民国三十七年二月
二十九日上海市医师公会颁发给陆坤豪的感谢
状，以谢忱陆先生对该会的热心捐助。文末钤
上海市医师公会图章和图记各一枚。已残破。
1955 年入藏。

中华医学会 / 上海中医药大学医史博物馆藏

Letter of Thanks to Lu Kunhao From Shanghai Physician Union

Modern Times

27.6 cm×25.5 cm

This rectangular letter of appreciation was issued
in February 29 of the 37th year of the Republic of
China, by Shanghai Physician Union to Lu Kunhao,
to thank him for his warmhearted donation to
Shanghai Physician Union. In the end there are a
seal and a stamp of Shanghai Physician Union. It
was collected in 1955 and has been incomplete.
Preserved in Chinese Medical Association/Museum
of Chinese Medicine, Shanghai University of
Traditional Chinese Medicine

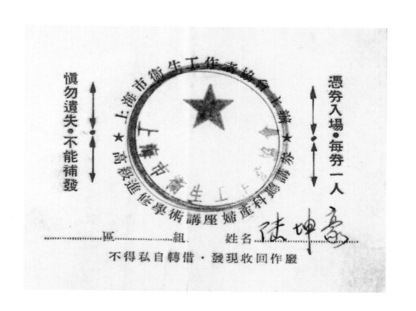

妇产科听讲券

近现代

9 厘米 ×7.3 厘米

纸卡形，为入场券。该藏用普通白纸铅印红字而成，加盖上海市卫生工作者协会蓝色图章，票面注明"高级进修学术讲座妇产科听讲券上海市卫生工作者协会主办陆坤豪"等字样。保存完好。1955 年入藏。

中华医学会 / 上海中医药大学医史博物馆藏

Admission Ticket of Gynaecology and Obstetrics Lecture

Modern Times

9 cm×7.3 cm

The document was printed with red characters in a normal white paper in lead print, with blue seal of Shanghai Association of Health Workers. There are characters meaning that it is an admission ticket of Gynaecology and Obstetrics Lecture hosted by Shanghai Association of Health Workers. The name Lu Kunhao was also on the ticket. It was collected in 1955 and is preserved well.

Preserved in Chinese Medical Association/Museum of Chinese Medicine, Shanghai University of Traditional Chinese Medicine

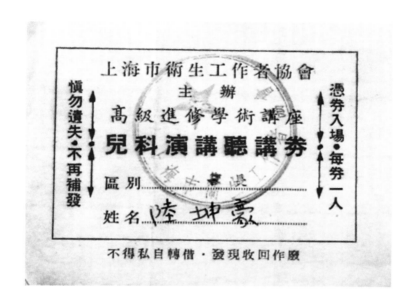

儿科演讲听讲券

近现代

9 厘米 ×6.7 厘米

纸卡形，为入场券。该藏用普通白纸铅印红字而成，加盖上海市卫生工作者协会蓝色图章，票面注明"高级进修学术讲座儿科演讲听讲券上海市卫生工作者协会主办陆坤豪"等字样。保存完好。保存完好。1955 年入藏。

中华医学会 / 上海中医药大学医史博物馆藏

Admission Ticket of Pediatrics Lecture

Modern Times

9 cm×6.7 cm

This admission ticket was printed with red characters in a normal white paper in lead print, with blue seal of Shanghai Association of Health Workers. There are characters meaning that it is an admission ticket of Pediatrics Lecture hosted by Shanghai Association of Health Workers. The name Lu Kunhao was also on the ticket. It was collected in 1955 and is preserved well.

Preserved in Chinese Medical Association/Museum of Chinese Medicine, Shanghai University of Traditional Chinese Medicine

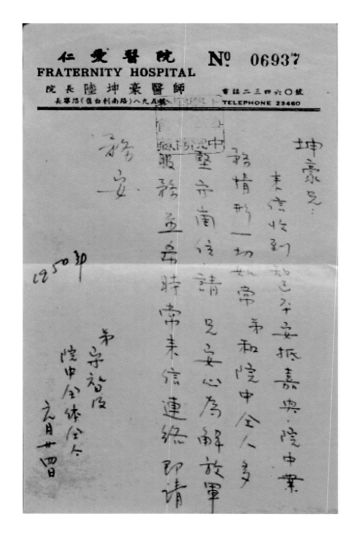

仁爱医院同仁致陆坤豪院长便函

近现代

19 厘米 ×10.5 厘米

Informal Letter of Colleagues of Charity Hospital To Dean Lu Kunhao

Modern Times

19 cm×10.5 cm

长方形，为信函。该藏用仁爱医院便笺纸书
就，是陆坤豪医师赴嘉兴为中国人民解放军
医治日本住血吸虫病期间，其弟陆守智代表
全院同仁于 1950 年 6 月 24 日给陆坤豪所写
便函。保存完好。1955 年入藏。

中华医学会 / 上海中医药大学医史博物馆藏

This letter was written on the rectangular
scribbling paper of Charity Hospital on June
24, 1950, by Lu Shouzhi, Lu Kunhao's little
brother, on behalf of all the colleagues of this
hospital, during the period when he was treating
schistosoma japonicum for Peoples Liberation
Army in Jianxing County, Zhejiang Province. It
was collected in 1955 and is preserved well.
Preserved in Chinese Medical Association/
Museum of Chinese Medicine, Shanghai
University of Traditional Chinese Medicine

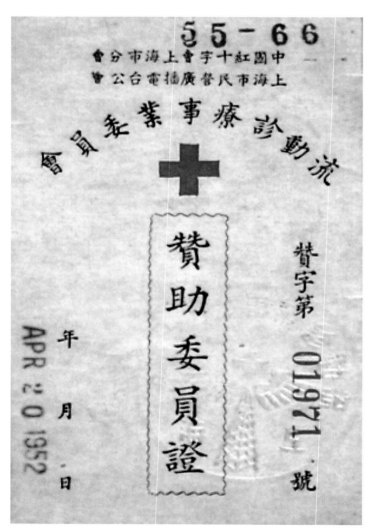

陆坤豪赞助委员证

近现代

9.4 厘米 ×5.7 厘米

Donation Certificate of Lun Kunhao

Modern Times

9.4 cm×5.7 cm

卡片式，为证件。该藏呈普通卡片式，铅印，正面有"中国红十字会上海市分会上海市民营广播电台公会流动诊疗事业委员会赞助委员证"，并注编号与日期；背面注明陆坤豪先生捐款事宜和证件使用规则。该藏钤"上海流动诊疗事业委员会"钢印。保存完好。1955 年入藏。

中华医学会 / 上海中医药大学医史博物馆藏

This document was printed in the rectangular card, with the characters on the cover showing the units like Shanghai Red Cross, Shanghai Private Broadcasting Union and Floating Treatment Experiment Committee as well as the name of the certificate with the number and date. The back shows the donation details of Mr. Lu and the usage of the certificate. It was collected in 1955 and is preserved well.

Preserved in Chinese Medical Association/ Museum of Chinese Medicine, Shanghai University of Traditional Chinese Medicine

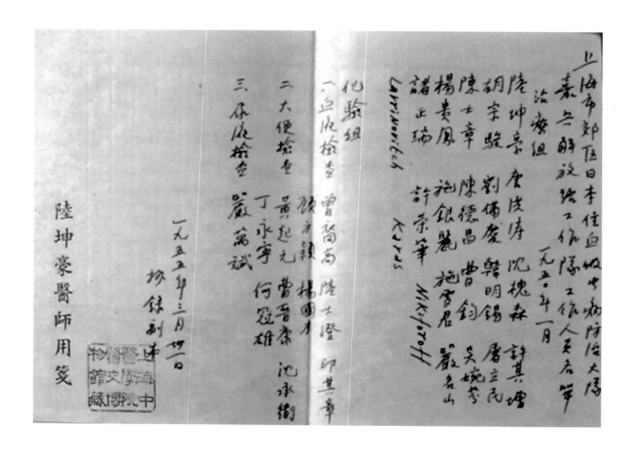

上海赴嘉兴血防队名单

近现代

19.4 厘米 ×13.5 厘米

Name List of Schistosoma Japonicum Control Group from Shanghai to Jiaxing

Modern Times

19.4 cm×13.5 cm

长方形，为名单录。钢笔书写于陆坤豪医师用笺上，内容是"上海郊区日本住血吸虫病防治大队嘉兴解放路工作队工作人员名单"，其人员分为治疗组和化验组共 32 人，其中有 3 名外国人。该藏是 1955 年 3 月 31 日抄录的副本。保存完好。1955 年入藏。

中华医学会 / 上海中医药大学医史博物馆藏

This collection was written with a fountain pen on the rectangular note-paper of Physician Lu Kunhao. It is the name list of members of the team in Jiefang Road, Jiaxing City, belonging to Schistosoma Japonicum Control Group in Shanghai suburbs. There were 32 members, divided into the treatment group and the test group, including three foreigners. This paper is a copied version on March 31, 1955. It was collected in 1955 and is preserved well.

Preserved in Chinese Medical Association/ Museum of Chinese Medicine, Shanghai University of Traditional Chinese Medicine

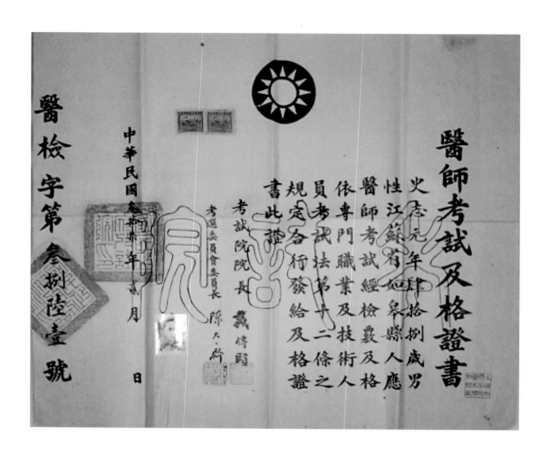

史志元医师考试及格证书

近现代

42.6 厘米 ×39.1 厘米

Physician Examination Pass Certificate of Shi Zhiyuan

Modern Times

42.6 cm×39.1 cm

长方形，为合格证书。该藏是民国三十七年二月国民政府考试院颁发给史志元中医师的考试及格证书，证书上方印有国民党党徽，并粘印花税票两张，价值1000元，下端粘有史志元照片，并钤钢印和国民政府考试院院长和考选委员会委员长的落款与钤记，末尾和骑缝钤有国民政府考试院印。保存基本完好。1955年入藏。

中华医学会/上海中医药大学医史博物馆藏

This document is a certificate issued by the Examination Council of the Republic of China to TCM Physician Shi Zhiyuan in November of the 37th year of the Republic of China. On the upper part there was the printed emblem of Kuo Min Tang, with two revenue stamps pasted on it, worth 100 yuan in total value. On the lower part, Shi's photo was pasted, with embossment and the signatures of the President of the Examination Council of the National Government and the Chairman of Selection Committee and seals. The seal of the Examination Council of the Republic of China can be seen in the end and on the perforation. It was collected in 1955 and is basically preserved well.

Preserved in Chinese Medical Association/Museum of Chinese Medicine, Shanghai University of Traditional Chinese Medicine

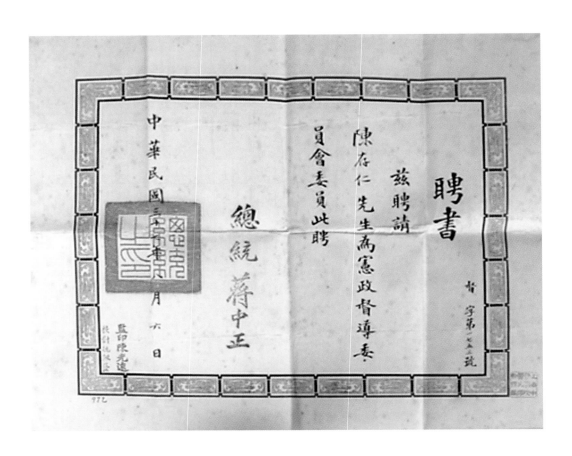

陈存仁聘书

近现代

46 厘米 ×36.9 厘米

Letter of Appointment of Chen Cunren

Modern Times

46 cm×36.9 cm

长方形，为聘书。该藏为中华民国三十七年八月六日
总统聘请陈存仁先生为"宪政督导委员会委员"的聘
书，文末有总统蒋中正落款和"总统之印"钤记。陈
存仁，上海人，毕业于上海中医专门学校，善内科、
妇科及针灸科，曾任上海市国民政府参议员及国大代
表，1949年去香港行医，后移居美国。保存完好。
1958年入藏。

中华医学会/上海中医药大学医史博物馆藏

This rectangular letter of appointment shows that on
August 6 of the 37th year of the Republic of China,
the President appointed Chen Cunren as a member of
Constitutional Supervision Committee. In the end, there
are the signature of Jiang Zhongzheng and his seal.
Chen Cunren was born in Shanghai. He graduated from
Shanghai College of Traditional Chinese Medicine,
and was good at Internal Medicine, Gynaecology, and
Acupuncture. He once was a senator of the National
Government in Shanghai and a representative of the
Congress Party. In 1949, he went to Hong Kang as a
physician. Later he moved to America. It was collected in
1958 and is preserved well.
Preserved in Chinese Medical Association/Museum of
Chinese Medicine, Shanghai University of Traditional
Chinese Medicine

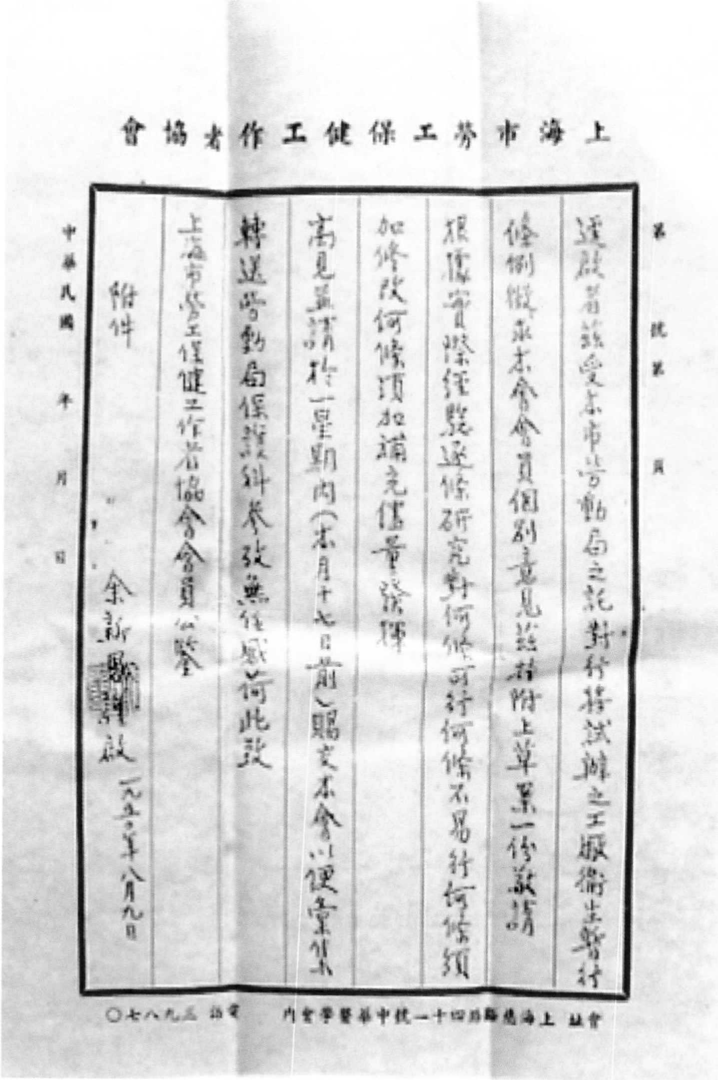

上海市勞工保健工作者協會

第　號第　頁

逕啟者茲受本市勞動局之託對於擬試辦之工廠衛生暫行
條例徵求本會會員個別意見茲將附上草案一份敬請
根據實際經驗逐條研究對何條可行何條不易行何條須
加修改何條須加補充儘量發揮
高見並請於一星期內（本月十七日前）賜交本會以便彙集
轉送勞動局保護科參考無任感荷此致
上海市勞工保健工作者協會會員台鑒
附件
余新恩敬 一九五三年八月九日

中華民國　年　月　日

會址 上海慈谿路四十一號中華醫學會內　電話 三九八七〇

余新恩函笺

近现代

27.2 厘米 ×19.1 厘米

Formal Letter by Yu Xin’en

Modern Times

27.2 cm×19.1 cm

长方形，为函笺。该藏用上海市劳工保健工作者协会函笺纸油印，内容为余新恩受市劳动局委托，就《工厂卫生暂行条例》（草案）征求意见事，发给上海市劳工保健工作者协会会员的函笺，行末有余新恩落款并钤印。保存基本完好。1955 年入藏。

中华医学会 / 上海中医药大学医史博物馆藏

This collection was written on the letter paper of Shanghai Labor Health Association. Commissioned by the Shanghai Municipal Labor Bureau, Yu Xin'en wrote this formal letter to members of Shanghai Labor Health Association, looking for advice towards the Draft of Interim Regulations on Factory's Healthy Working Environment. In the end, there are his signature and personal seal. It was collected in 1955 and is preserved well.

Preserved in Chinese Medical Association/ Museum of Chinese Medicine, Shanghai University of Traditional Chinese Medicine

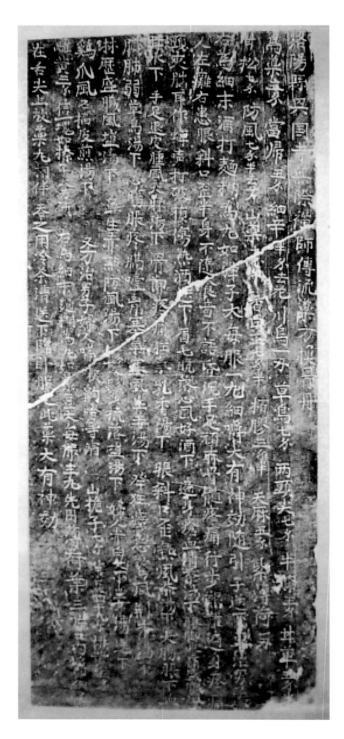

换骨丹药方碑拓

近现代

长 76.5 厘米，宽 31 厘米

Stone Tablet Rubbing of *Huan Gu Dan Yao Fang*

Modern Times

Length 76.5 cm/ Width 31 cm

长方形，药方碑拓。原碑立于宋代洛阳兴国
寺，内容为该寺无际禅师所传治疗骨科疾病
之换骨丹等药方。保存完好。

中华医学会 / 上海中医药大学医史博物馆藏

Huan Gu Dan Yao Fang is literally translated as
"the prescriptions for treating bone diseases".
The tablet was rectangular. The original tablet
was placed in Xingguo Temple in Luo Yang
City in the Song Dynasty. The content of the
tablet was about the prescriptions of medicines
that were used by a Zen Master named Wu Ji.
The rubbing is well preserved.
Preserved in Chinese Medical Association/
Museum of Chinese Medicine, Shanghai
University of Traditional Chinese Medicine

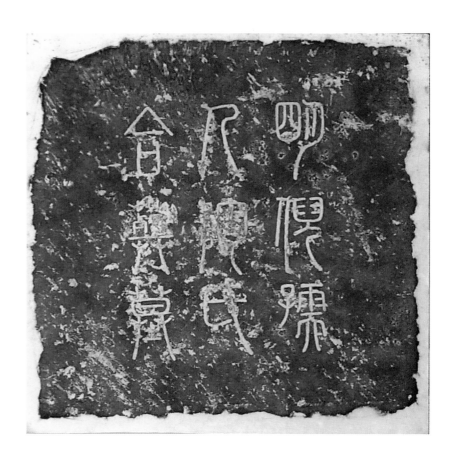

明倪儒人陶氏合葬墓志铭文石刻拓片

近现代

长 56.3 厘米，宽 54.7 厘米

Rubbing of the Multi-burial Tombstone of the Ni Ru Ren and Tao

Modern Times

Length 56.3 cm/ Width 54.7 cm

长方形，为碑拓。该石刻在上海南汇发现，共两块，一为篆刻大字"明倪儒人陶氏合葬墓"石刻，一为楷书小字墓志铭内容，据专家考证内有针刺治疗白内障的记载，前后均为明代江南四大才子之一文徵明晚年珍迹。倪儒人详情待考。该藏为大字拓片。保存完好，文字模糊。

中华医学会/上海中医药大学医史博物馆藏

The original stone tablets were found in Nanhui, Shanghai, one of which was inscribed "Ming Ni Ru Ren Tao Shi He Zang Mu" (the multi-burial tomb of Ni Ru Ren and Tao in the Ming Dynasty) and another was inscribed with the epitaph in small standard script of handwriting. The content of the epitome, after textual research by experts, was about treatment cataract with acupuncture and was written by Wen Zhengming (one of the four great southern talents of the Ming Dynasty). Details about Ni Ru Ren remain to be found out. The picture shown above was the large-character rubbing of the stone tablet, which is preserved well with blurred characters.

Preserved in Chinese Medical Association/Museum of Chinese Medicine, Shanghai University of Traditional Chinese Medicine

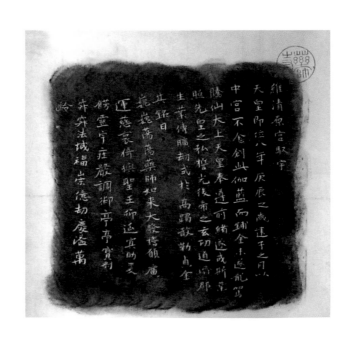

天皇铭药师寺拓片

近现代

画芯长 43.2 厘米，宽 42.2 厘米

卷轴，为碑拓。拓片除碑刻楷书文字外，还有篆体圆印"药师之印"钤记。碑刻其他情况待考。保存基本完好，已装裱成卷轴，画面有污迹。1960 年入藏。

中华医学会／上海中医药大学医史博物馆藏

Stone Rubbing from Yakushi-ji Made by Emperor Tenmu

Modern Times

Length 43.2 cm/ Width 42.2 cm

This collection is a rubbing. Apart from characters in regular script engraved on the stone, there is also a stamp of "Yao Shi Zhi Yin" (Pharmacist's seal) in seal characters. Other information on the stone remains to be verified. It is preserved well. It has been made into scroll with some stains on it. It was collected in 1960.

Preserved in Chinese Medical Association/Museum of Chinese Medicine, Shanghai University of Traditional Chinese Medicine

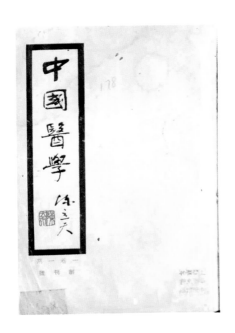

《中国医学》杂志创刊号

近现代

27.1 厘米 ×19.5 厘米

1937 年 7 月在上海创刊 ,8 月停刊 , 共出 2 期。

上海中医药博物馆藏

First Issue of *Zhong Guo Yi Xue*

Modern Times

27.1 cm×19.5 cm

The journal "Zhong Guo Yi xue" (*Chinese Medicine*) was started in Shanghai in July 1937. It was discontinued in August 1937. There were totally two issues published.

Preserved in Shanghai Museum of Traditional Chinese Medicine

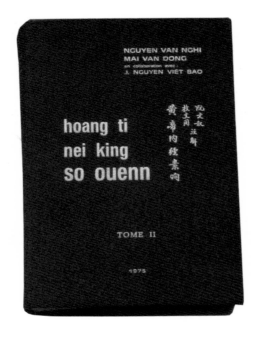

《黄帝内经·素问》（英文本）

近现代

25.4 厘米 ×17.3 厘米

书本形，为医籍。《黄帝内经·素问》（英文本）译著者为雅各布 W·林道，以《黄帝内经》京口文成堂摹刻宋本译出。保存完好。

中华医学会／上海中医药大学医史博物馆藏

Hoang Ti Nei King (English Version)

Modern Times

25.4 cm×17.3 cm

This medical classic Hoang *Ti Nei King* So Duenn (English Version) was translated by Tacob W · Lindau who adopted the Song Dynasty edition of Wencheng Tang in Jing Kou. It is preserved well. Preserved in Chinese Medical Association/Museum of Chinese Medicine, Shanghai University of Traditional Chinese Medicine

《本草纲目》（法文本）

近现代

23.2 厘米 ×17.5 厘米

书本形，为医籍。该藏本为 20 世纪初出版，为节译本，出版者待考。保存基本完好，纸张泛黄，局部磨损。

中华医学会 / 上海中医药大学医史博物馆藏

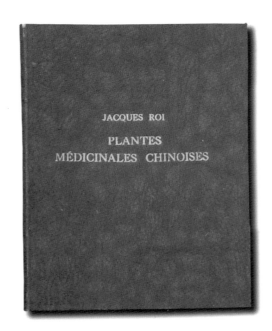

Plantes Medicinales Chinoises (French Version)

Modern Times

23.2 cm×17.5 cm

This collection was published in early 20th century. It is a selected translation version. The publisher remains to be proven. It is well preserved with yellow discolouration. Some parts of it have abrasions.

Preserved in Chinese Medical Association/Museum of Chinese Medicine, Shanghai University of Traditional Chinese Medicine

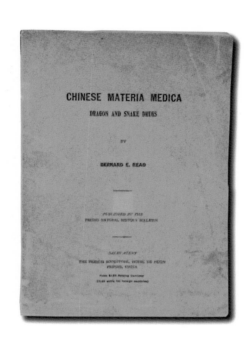

《本草纲目》（英文本）

近现代

25.8 厘米 ×18.3 厘米

书本形，为医籍。该藏本为 20 世纪初出版，为节译本，伯纳德 E·里德译，*THE PEIKING NATURAL HISTORY BULLETIN* 出版。保存基本完好，纸张泛黄，局部磨损。

中华医学会 / 上海中医药大学医史博物馆藏

Chinese Materia Medica (English Version)

Modern Times

25.8 cm×18.3 cm

This collection was published in early 20th century. It is a selected translation version. It was translated by Bernard E. Read, and published by the Peiking Natural History Bulletin. It is basically well-preserved with yellow discolouration. Some parts of it have abrasions.

Preserved in Chinese Medical Association/Museum of Chinese Medicine, Shanghai University of Traditional Chinese Medicine

《本草纲目》（英文本）

近现代

25.8 厘米 ×18.3 厘米

书本形，为医籍。该藏本为 1936 年伊博恩博士和刘汝强先生合作的《中华植物考》之一，北京出版，书名亦译作《本草新注》。保存基本完好，纸张泛黄，局部磨损。

　　中华医学会 / 上海中医药大学医史博物馆藏

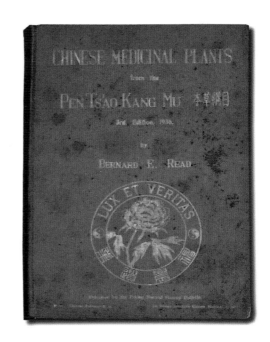

Chinese Medical Plants (English Version)

Modern Times

25.8 cm×18.3 cm

This collection was one of the Chinese botanic investigations made by Dr. Iborn and Mr. Liu Ruqiang in 1936. It was published in Beijing, and also called *Ben Cao Xin Zhu* (The New Annotated Compendium of Materia Medica). It is basically well preserved with yellow discolouration. Some parts of it have abrasions.

Preserved in Chinese Medical Association/Museum of Chinese Medicine, Shanghai University of Traditional Chinese Medicine

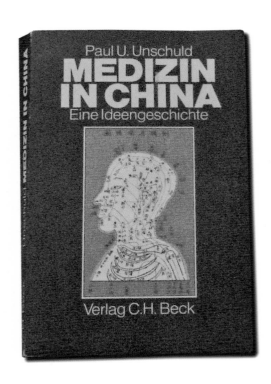

《中国医学》（德文本）

近现代

22.9 厘米 ×14.1 厘米

书本形，为医籍。《中国医学》（德文本）译著
者为德国慕尼黑大学文树德教授。全书 336 页，
1980 年由德国出版。保存完好。

中华医学会 / 上海中医药大学医史博物馆藏

Medizin in China (German Version)

Modern Times

22.9 cm×14.1 cm

The book was translated by Professor Paul
U. Unschuld at University of Munich. There were
totally 336 pages. The book was published in
German in 1980. It is well preserved.

Preserved in Chinese Medical Association/Museum
of Chinese Medicine, Shanghai University of
Traditional Chinese Medicine

《中国医学》（英文本）

近现代

25.5 厘米 ×17.3 厘米

书本形，为医籍。《中国医学》（英文本）译著
者为德国慕尼黑大学文树德教授。全书 403 页，
1990 年由美国出版。保存完好。

中华医学会 / 上海中医药大学医史博物馆藏

Forgotten Traditions of Ancient Chinese Medicine (English Version)

Modern

25.5 cm×17.3 cm

It is a book-shaped medical classic. It was translated
by Professor Paul U. Unschuld at University of
Munich. There were totally 403 pages. The book
was published in America in 1990. It is well
preserved.

Preserved in Chinese Medical Association/Museum
of Chinese Medicine, Shanghai University of
Traditional Chinese Medicine

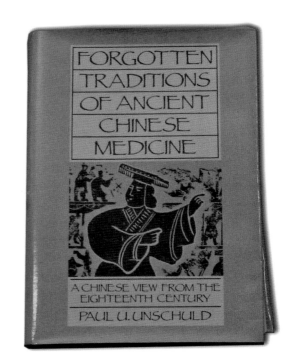

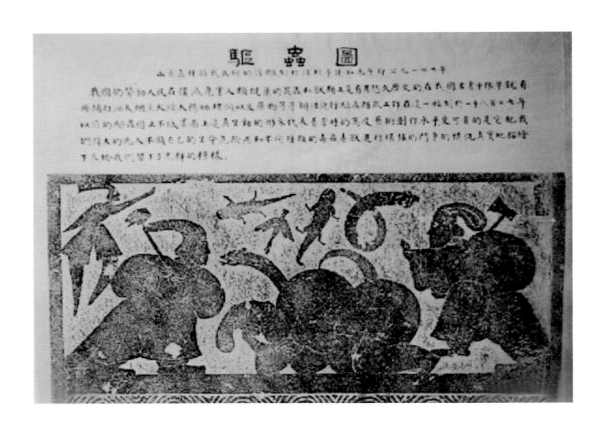

驱虫图

近现代

60 厘米 ×50 厘米

Painting of Expelling Parasite

Modern Times

60 cm×50 cm

山东嘉祥县吴氏祠的浮雕，刻于汉桓帝建和元年即公元 147 年，反映了我国劳动人民扑灭危害人类健康的昆虫和兽类的历史。画面形象、生动、逼真，代表当时高超的艺术水平。我国古书很早就有用捕打、洒灰、烟熏、火燎、太阳晒、堵洞及药物等方法驱虫、防虫的记载。

广东中医药博物馆藏

It is the embossment at Wu Shi Ci (name of an ancestral hall) in Jiaxiang County, Shandong Province. It was made in the first year of the reign of Emperor Huandi in the Han Dynasty (147). It shows the history of Chinese working people eliminating harmful insects and beasts. The vivid image shows the superb artistic level at that time. In ancient books, there were insect-resistant methods such as slapping, ashing, smudging, burning, drying in the sun, plugging, and drug.

Preserved in Guangdong Chinese Medicine Museum

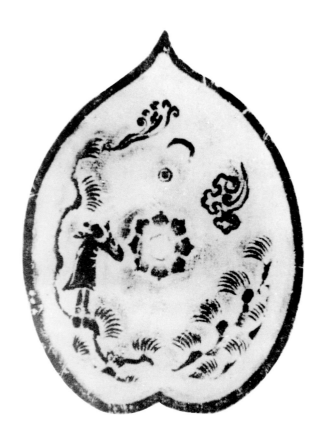

观星望月气功纹铜镜拓本

近现代

长 13.4 厘米

铜镜为宋代。镜为桃形，花瓣钮座。钮上云朵中有半月星辰，钮下草丛中站立一人，全神贯注，观星望月，正在做气功。

湖南省博物馆藏

Rubbing of Copper Mirror of Observing Constellations

Modern Times

Length 13.4 cm

The mirror in the Song Dynasty is peach-shaped, with a petal-like knob. There are cloud and constellations upon the knob. Under the knob, there is a person standing in the grass who concentrates on observing the constellations as well as doing "Qigong".

Preserved in Hunan Museum

龟咽鹤息气功纹铜镜拓本

近现代

边长 9.1 厘米

铜镜为宋代。方形，圆钮。钮座外一树虬曲绕钮
座，右侧上方有一展翅飞翔的仙鹤，下方有一龟
在伸颈吐气，左侧一人拱手遥望飞鹤，在做气功。

湖南省博物馆藏

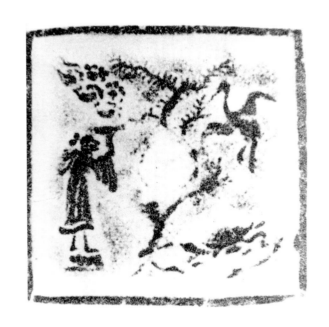

Rubbing of Copper Mirror of Tortoise and Crane

Modern Times

Side Length 9.1cm

The rubbing in the Song Dynasty is square and
has a round knob. Outside the knob, there is a tree
enclosing the knob. There is a crane at the right
side of the tree spreading its wings to fly. Under
the tree, there is a tortoise stretching its neck to
breathe. There is a person at the left side of the
tree submissively looking at the crane while doing
"Qigong".

Preserved in Hunan Museum

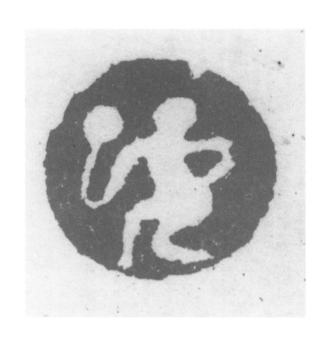

拍球纹肖形印拓本

近现代

直径 0.9 厘米

印为汉代。印面圆形，图案中一人曲腿、弓腰，其右臂上方雕一球，表示的应是拍球活动中的一个动作瞬间。

陈介祺《十钟山房印举》著录

Seal Rubbing of Bouncing the Ball

Modern Times

Diameter 0.9 cm

This stone rubbing was maed in the Han Dynasty. The round-shaped seal surface is carved with a person who bends his leg and waist, with his hand holding a ball, which vividly depicts the moment of action.

Recorded in *Shi Zhong Shan Fang Yin Ju* written by Chen Jieqi

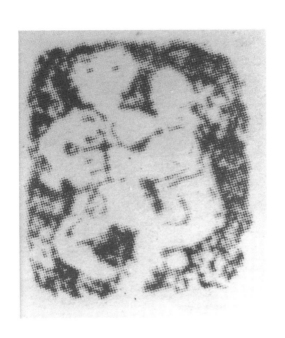

角抵纹肖形印拓本

近现代

长 1.4 厘米，宽 1 厘米

印为汉代铜质，印面长方形。印纹中两摔跤者正互相搂抱在一起，显得难分难解，表现了双方激战中扣人心弦的一瞬间。

故宫博物院藏

Seal Rubbing of Jue Di (Ancient Wrestling)

Modern Times

Length 1.4 cm/ Width 1 cm

The rectangular seal was made in the Han Dynasty. Its surface is carved with two wrestlers who grapple with each other and are locked in the battle, vividly depicting an exciting moment in the fierce fight.

Preserved in the Palace Museum

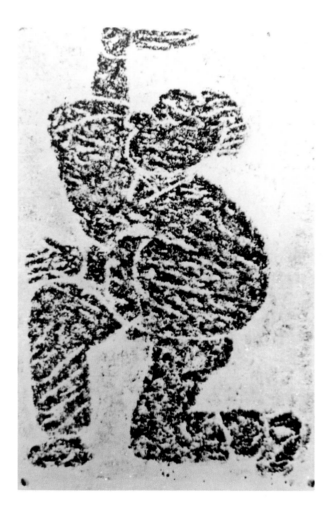

力士画像石拓本

近现代

长 70 厘米，宽 45 厘米

原画像为汉代。画面中力士散发，着上衣，一手置于胸前，一手托举，左腿跪地. 似有千斤之力。河南省唐河县电厂出土。

河南省南阳市唐河县博物馆藏

Stone Rubbing of Chinese Hercules

Modern Times

Length 70 cm/ Width 45 cm

The stone was made in the Han Dynasty. The hercules in the stone relief wears coat, with hair disheveled. He puts one hand over his chest, raises another and kneels down on his left knee, as if he has infinite strength. It was unearthed from the electric power plant in Tanghe County, Henan Province.

Preserved in Tanghe County Museum, Hanyang City, Henan Province

蹶张画像石拓本

近现代

长 68 厘米，宽 56 厘米

原画像石为汉代。蹶张头戴平帻，身着短衣，口
衔一矢，双脚踏弓，两手奋力张弦，似有臂张千
弓之力。河南省唐河县电厂出土。

河南省南阳市唐河县博物馆藏

Stone Rubbing of Jue Zhang

Modern Times

Length 68 cm/ Width 56 cm

The stone was made in the Han Dynasty. With flat
turban and short coat, Jue Zhang bites an arrow in
the mouth, steps on the bow and exerts himself to
pull back the cord, as if he had infinite power. The
stone was unearthed from the electric power plant
in Tanghe County, Henan Province.

Preserved in Tanghe County Museum, Nanyang
City, Henan Province

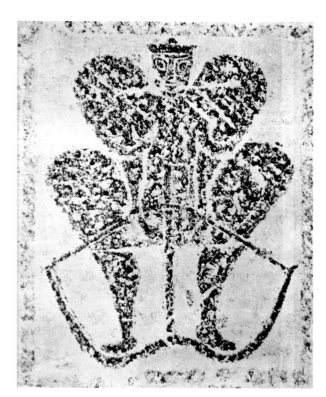

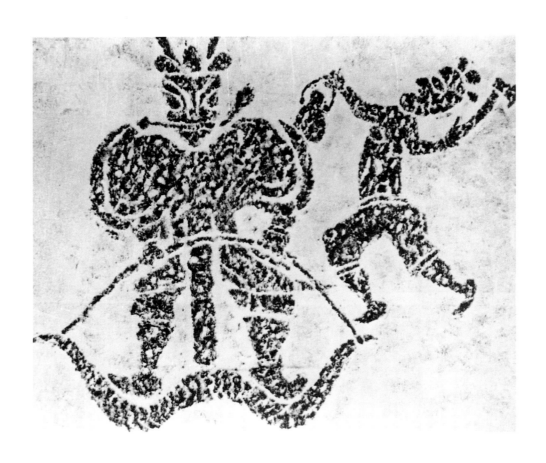

蹶张画像石拓本

近现代

长 106 厘米，宽 86 厘米

Stone Rubbing of Jue Zhang

Modern Times

Length 106 cm/ Width 86 cm

原画像石为汉代。蹶张，为足踏强弓练力之武士。画面中的蹶张，口衔一矢，两脚踏弓，奋力张弦，显示出强犬的力量。其右刻一人，一手持斧，一手提壶。河南省唐河县湖阳辛店出土。

河南省南阳市唐河县博物馆藏

The stone was made in the Han Dynasty. Jue Zhang is a warrior who steps on the bow to tone up the muscles. In the picture, he bites an arrow in the mouth, steps on the bow, and exerts himself to pull back the cord, demonstrating his great power. On the right of Jue Zhang is a person, who holds an axe in one hand and a pot in another. The stone was unearthed in Xindian Village, Huyang Town, Tanghe County, Henan Province.

Preserved in Tanghe County Museum, Nanyang City, Henan Province

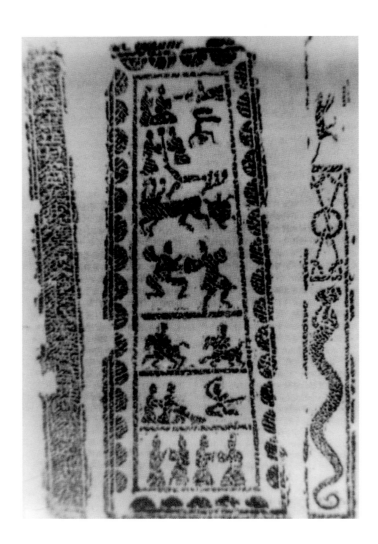

拳术对搏画像石拓本

近现代
长 180 厘米，宽 52~70 厘米

Stone Rubbing of Chinese Boxing

Modern
Length 180 cm/ Width 52–70 cm

原画像石为东汉。此石为阙身，呈梯形。画面共分四层：二层，两骑者；三层，舞乐；四层，四人对揖；而第一层，除了人物拜谒、倒立伎和多头人面兽外，主要内容就是徒手对搏形象。对搏的两人均赤手，头束发髻，上着紧腰衣，下穿紧身裤，作蹲步、弓腰，正在伺机向对方进攻，这应是武术中较早的拳术技击形式。1965 年山东省莒南县东汉孙氏墓出土。

山东省博物馆藏

The stone was made in the Eastern Han Dynasty. The ladder-shaped stone seems like a watchtower. The relief consists of four layers. On the second floor are two riders, and on the third floor are dancer and singer. In the fourth floor are four people making bows with hands folded in front, while the top part of the picture is carved with bare-handed Chinese boxing game, in which two boxers, with hairs in buns and tight-fitting clothe and pants, squat on the heels and bend their waists, watching for chances to attack each other, which is an early form of Chines boxing arts of attack and defense. It was unearthed from Sun's Tomb of Eastern Han Dynasty in Junan County, Shandong Province, in 1965.

Preserved in Shandong Museum

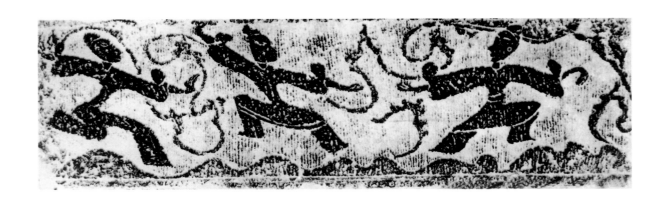

拳勇画像石拓本

近现代

长 136 厘米，宽 44 厘米

原画像为东汉。图中共三人，右边二人均呈马步，伸掌欲击向对方，左边一人似在旁边指点什么，当为裁判一类的人物。

河南省南阳汉画馆藏

Stone Rubbing of Chinese Boxing

Modern Times

Length 136 cm/ Width 44 cm

The stone was made in Eastern Han Dynasty. It is carved with three people, among which two keep horse stance and shake their fists to hit each other. The person in the left gives directions to them as judge.

Preserved in Nanyang Stone-carved art Museum in Han Dynasty

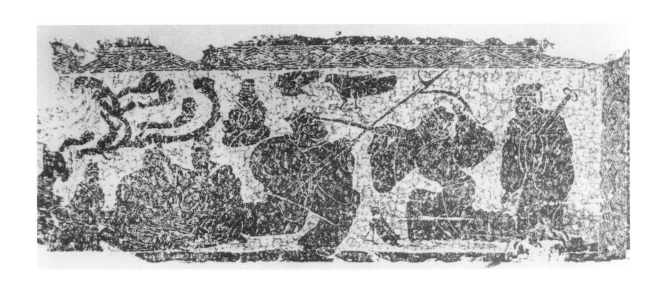

比武画像石拓本

近现代

长 151 厘米，宽 95 厘米

此画像石为汉代。图中左边一人手持长戟，弓步前刺；右边一人左手执钩镶，右手持剑相迎，动态美而矫健。旁有几位观者。1956 年江苏省铜山县苗山出土。

徐州汉画像石艺术馆藏

Stone Rubbing of Competition in Military Skills

Modern Times

Length 151 cm/ Width 95 cm

The stone was made in the Eastern Han Dynasty. In the left part of the relief is a person, holding a long halberd, who lunges forward to thrust. In the right part, a person holds Gouxiang (an ancient shield-like weapon) in the left hand and defends himself with the sword in the right hand. Surrounding two fighters are some spectators. It was unearthed in Miaoshan Mountain in Tongshan County, Jiangsu Province，in 1956.

Preserved in Xuzhou Museum of Paintings and Stone Arts in Han Dynasty

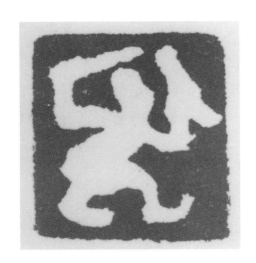

执刀盾肖形印拓本

近现代

边长 1 厘米

此为汉代执刀盾肖形印的拓本。印为铜质，印面呈正方形，所刻图案为一左手执盾、右手持刀的武士，正弓腰技击。

上海博物馆藏

Rubbing of Pictorial Seal Carved with Warrior

Modern Times

Side Length 1 cm

This is a rubbing of a pictorial bronze seal. The surface of the square seal was carved with a warrior who holds a shield in the left hand and a knife in the right hand. He bends down and gets ready to fight.

Preserved in Shanghai Museum

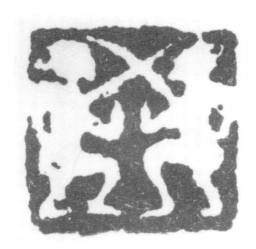

执刀技击肖形印拓本

近现代

边长 1 厘米

此为汉代执刀技击肖形印的拓本。印面呈正方形，图案刻有二武士，正各执一刀做出相互技击之状。

殷康辑《古图形玺印汇》著录

Rubbing of Pictorial Seal Carved with Martial Arts

Modern Times

Side Length 1 cm

This is a rubbing of a pictorial seal carved with martial arts. The surface of the square seal was carved with two warriors, each holding a knife, ready to attack each other.

Recorded in *Collection of Ancient Graphic Seals* by Yin Kang

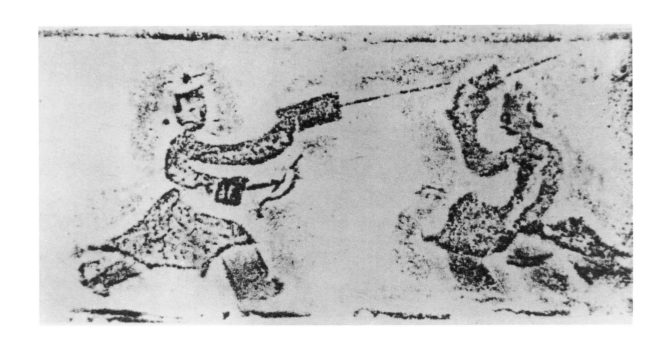

击剑画像砖拓本

近现代

长 10.4 厘米，宽 5.8 厘米

Brick Rubbing of Fencing

Modern Times

Length 10.4 cm/ Width 5.8 cm

原画像砖为汉代。画面中两个头戴冠、身着长衣的武士在进行击剑对刺。左边的人左手持剑，上弓步直刺，同时右手持钩镶前伸准备防御；右边的人左手持钩镶，右手挑剑，面对对方刺来的剑，正在躲闪防御。河南省郑州市出土。

河南博物院藏

The stone was made in the Han Dynasty. In the relief are two warriors who are fencing, wearing hats and tunics. The person on the left, holding sword in his left hand, lunges forward to thrust, and defends himself with Gouxiang (an ancient shield-like weapon). The person on the right is protecting himself from the attack from the left one, holding up his sword in the right hand and taking Gouxiang in the left one. It was unearthed in Zhengzhou City, Henan Province.

Preserved in Henan Museum

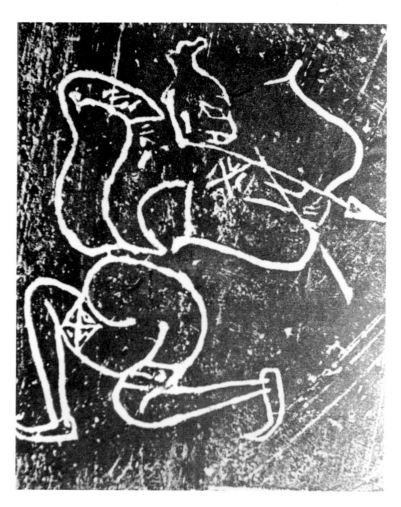

跪射画像砖拓本

近现代

长 25 厘米，宽 18 厘米

Brick Rubbing of Kneeling Archer

Modern Times

Length 25 cm/ Width 18 cm

原画像砖为西汉。画面上，一戴帻猎人著带边饰上衣短绔，跨弓步跪地，侧转上身奋力拉弓，动势、表情十分生动形象。河南省洛阳市东赵出土。

河南博物院藏

The brick in the Western Han Dynasty is carved with a hunter who wears turban, shorts and clothes with edging. He lunges forward, kneels down and turns around, pulling the bow. The expression and action of the archer is vividly and lively depicted on the relief. It was unearthed in Dongzhao Village, Luoyang City, Henan Province.

Preseved in Henan Museum

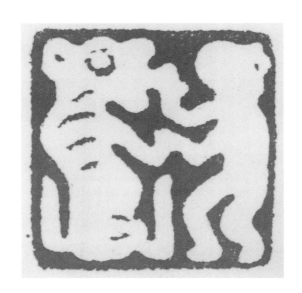

斗虎纹肖形印拓本

近现代

边长 1 厘米

印为汉代铜质。印面正方形。印纹中被斗之虎张开大口已有噬人之意，而斗虎者则一手抓住虎的一只前腿，另一手正举拳击向虎口，场面扣人心弦。

上海博物馆藏

Seal Rubbing of Tiger Fighter

Modern Times

Side Length 1 cm

The square seal was made in the Han Dynasty. The surface is carved with a tiger who opens its mouth and wants to swallow people while a fighter who grips one of tiger's legs in one hand and strikes another fist on its mouth, representing an exciting moment in fight.

Preserved in Shanghai Museum

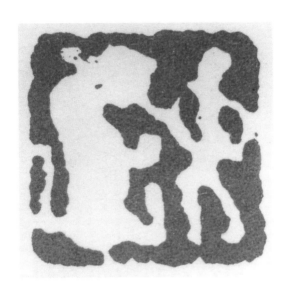

斗虎纹肖形印拓本

近现代

边长 1 厘米

印为汉代铜质。印面正方形。印纹刻画的是一武士在正面挑逗猛虎，被激怒的猛虎已有张牙舞爪欲搏噬人之意，但武士仍沉着与之嬉戏挑逗。孙壮辑《雪园藏印》（钤印本）著录。

中国国家图书馆藏

Seal Rubbing of Tiger Fighter

Modern Times

Side Length 1 cm

The square seal was made in the Han Dynasty. The surface is carved with a warrior who provokes the tiger on purpose. Though the fierce-looking tiger wants to eat him, he still keeps calm and plays with it. It is recorded in *Xue Yuan Cang Yin* (Seals in Snow Garden) by Sun Zhuangji.

Preserved in National Library of China

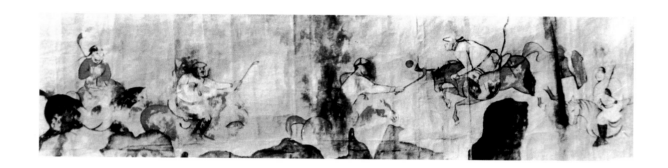

打马球图壁画摹本

近现代

原图长180厘米，宽50厘米

Facsimile of Mural Painting of Playing Polo

Modern Times

Length 180 cm/ Width 50 cm

原壁画绘 于辽代。打马球图位于墓室西壁。整
个画面自左至右共有 5 位竞技者在骑马挥杖击
球。图中人物的动作、服饰、所击之球及奔马的
形态，清晰可辨，反映出一场激烈的马球比赛正
在进行。1990 年内蒙古自治区敖汉旗宝国吐乡
皮匠沟辽代 1 号壁画墓出土。

敖汉旗博物馆藏

The mural painting of playing polo was made in
the Liao Dynasty. It is on the west wall of coffin
chamber. From left to right in the picture are five
competitors on the horses, swinging at the ball.
The action and the clothes of the riders, the ball
and the posture of running horses, which are all
vividly depicted in the picture, represent an exciting
game. It was unearthed from the No. 1 Tomb in the
Liao Dynasty in Pijianggou in Baoguotu village,
Aohan banner, Inner Mongolia Autonomous
Region in 1990.

Preserved in Aohan Banner Museum

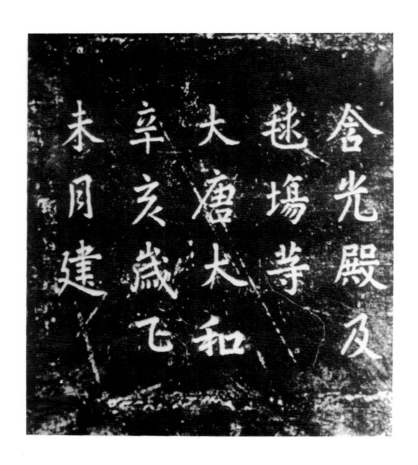

长安城大明宫含光殿石志拓本

近现代

长 53.5 厘米，宽 53.5 厘米

Rubbing of Stone Inscription in Hanguang Hall of Daming Palace

Modern Times

Length 53.5 cm/ Width 53.5 cm

此为唐代球场的石志拓本。石志发现于含光殿殿基下，方形。刻文位于石面中心："含光殿及球场等，大唐大和辛亥岁乙未建"。这一记述表明了唐文宗大和五年（831）十一月，在文明宫修建了"含光殿及球场等"。这是我们研究唐代体育活动场地的珍贵资料。1956 年陕西省西安市大明宫遗址出土。

中国国家博物馆藏

This is a rubbing of a stone inscription about the polo fields in the Tang Dynasty. The square stone was found under the base of Hanguang Hall, with inscription engraved in the center, recording that the hall and sports fields were both built in Xinhai year during the reign titled Dahe in the Tang Dynasty, to be exact, in November of the 5th year (A.D. 831) in the reign of Emperor Wenzong. The stone inscription is invaluable resource for us to research on the sports fields of the Tang Dynasty. It was unearthed in 1956 in the historic site of Daming Palace in Xi'an, Shaanxi Province.

Preserved in National Museum of China

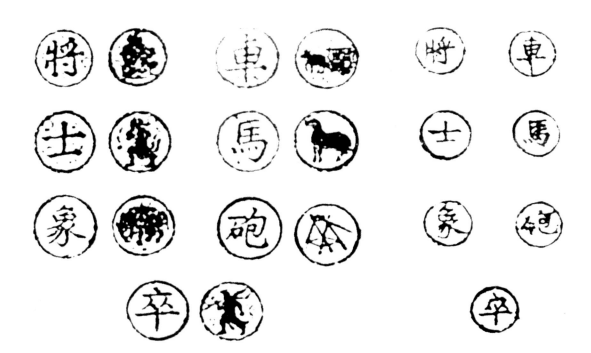

铜质象棋子拓本

近现代

直径 2.3~2.5 厘米，厚 0.2 厘米

Rubbing of Bronze Chinese Chess Pieces

Modern Times

Diameter 2.3-2.5 cm/ Thickness 0.2 cm

此为宋代铜质象棋子拓本，，共计 31 枚。棋子正面为阳书楷体汉字，背面为相应的图案，边缘有一穿孔。包括"将"二枚、"士"三枚、"象"四枚、"马"四枚、"车"四枚、"炮"四枚及"卒"十枚。1983 四川省江油县彰明公社出土。

绵阳市江油博物馆藏

This is a rubbing of 31 bronze Chinese Chess pieces, each of which is carved with a regular scrip in relief on the front and the corresponding pattern on the back, as well as one piercing at the rim. This set of Chinese chess includes two "commanders in chief", three "bodyguards", four "elephants", four "horses", two "chariots", four "cannons" and ten "pawns". These pieces of Chinese chess were unearthed in Zhangming Commune, Jiangyou County, Sichuan Province, in 1983.

Preserved in Jiangyou Museum, Mianyang City

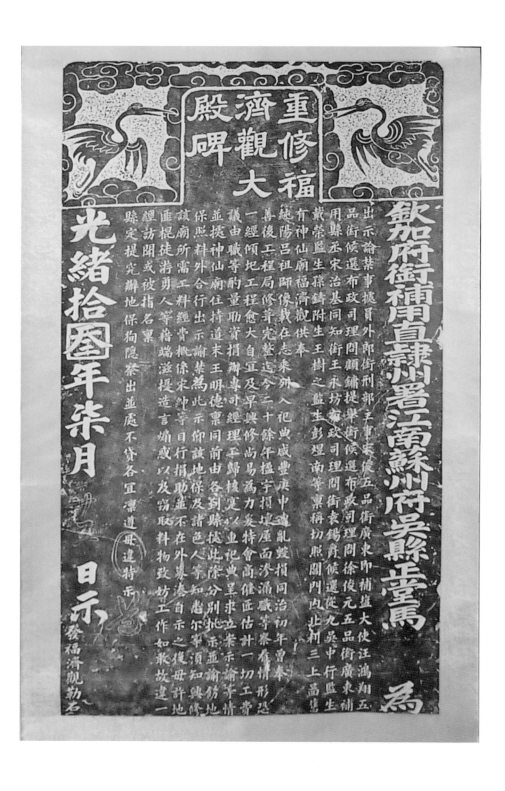

重修福济观大殿碑拓

近现代

卷轴：长 211.4 厘米，宽 72.6 厘米

画芯：长 129.1 厘米，宽 60.8 厘米

卷轴，是拓片。该碑记是光绪十三年重修福济观大殿时所刻。福济观在苏州吴县。碑拓已裱成卷轴，纸张泛黄，画面有污迹。1958 年入藏。

中华医学会 / 上海中医药大学医史博物馆藏

Stone Rubbing Inscription for Renovation of Main Hall in Fuji Temple

Modern Times

Scroll: Length 211.4 cm/ Width 72.6 cm

Picture: Length 129.1 cm/ Width 60.8 cm

The inscription was engraved on the stone during the renovation of main hall in Fuji Temple in the 13th year in the reign of Emperor Guangxu in Wuxian County, Suzhou City. Mounted into scroll, the rubbing has been faded and turned yellow, with some stains. It was collected in 1958.

Preserved in Chinese Medical Association/Museum of Chinese Medicine, Shanghai University of Traditional Chinese Medicine

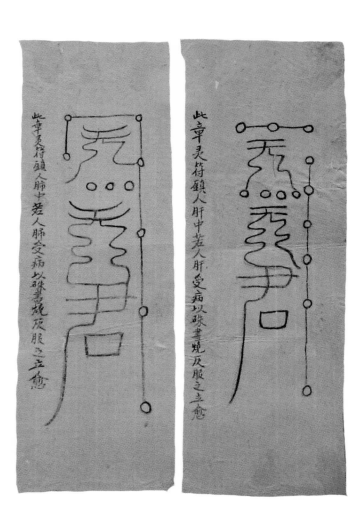

祛病灵符

近现代

左：24.3 厘米 ×7.8 厘米

右：24.7 厘米 ×8.3 厘米

Magic Figures for Eliminating Disease

Modern Times

Left: 24.3 cm ×7.8 cm

Right: 24.7 cm×8.3 cm

长方形，为巫术用品。该藏由两张长条形泛黄白纸黑墨书画而成。其中一张标有"此章灵符镇人肝中若人肝受病以硃书烧灰服之立愈"；另一张标有"此章灵符镇人肺中若人肺受病以硃书烧灰服之立愈"。保存基本完好，纸张泛黄。

中华医学会/上海中医药大学医史博物馆藏

These magic figures consist of two rectangular pictures with patterns in black ink on yellowing white paper, used for practicing witchcraft. The characters marked on these two figures record that one could cure liver disease when burnt into medicine powder with red paper, and another could cure lung diseases. These two magic figures are still in good condition with yellow discoloration.

Preserved in Chinese Medical Association/Museum of Chinese Medicine, Shanghai University of Traditional Chinese Medicine

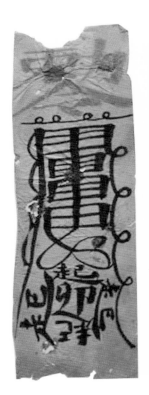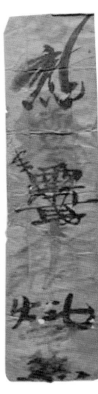

辟邪符

近现代

左：28.4 厘米 ×9 厘米

右：29.5 厘米 ×6.5 厘米

长方形，为辟邪用品。该藏由两张长条形泛黄白纸红黑墨书画而成，图案和字迹待考。保存基本完好，纸张泛黄。

中华医学会／上海中医药大学医史博物馆藏

Magic Figures for Counteracting Evil Force

Modern Times

Left: 28.4 cm ×9 cm

Right: 29.5 cm×6.5 cm

Used to counteract evil force, the magic figures consist of two rectangular pictures with patterns in red and black ink, while the diagram and characters remain to be verified. These two magic figures are still in good condition with yellow discoloration.

Preserved in Chinese Medical Association/Museum of Chinese Medicine, Shanghai University of Traditional Chinese Medicine

辟邪纸符

近现代

35.3 厘米 ×25.2 厘米

长方形，为辟邪用品。该藏用普通白纸粉彩绘就，画面绘有神鬼画像 11 个，中部莲花台托起一牌匾，上书"天地三界十方万灵真乐"字样。边缘破损。

中华医学会 / 上海中医药大学医史博物馆藏

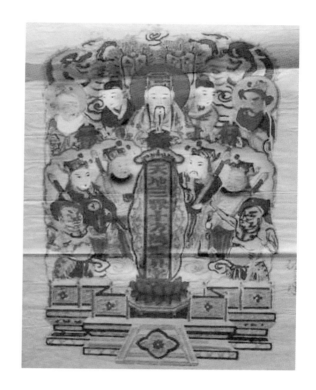

Magic Figure for Counteracting Evil Force

Modern Times

35.3 cm ×25.2 cm

Used to counteract evil force, the magic figure was painted on white paper in color ink. On the figure with edge-clipping are eleven supernatural images, holding a plaque which says "All the creatures in universe will enjoy happiness". The edges have been worn out.

Preserved in Chinese Medical Association/Museum of Chinese Medicine, Shanghai University of Traditional Chinese Medicine

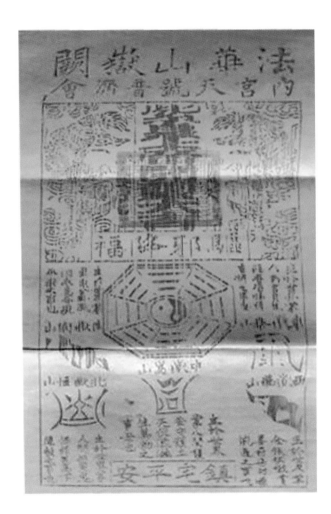

法华山镇宅符

近现代

43.5 厘米 ×20.5 厘米

**Magic Figure of Fahua Mountain
for Stabilizing the House**

Modern Times

43.5 cm×20.5 cm

长方形，为辟邪用品。该藏由普通白纸木刻板印制、装裱成镜片，上部印有"法华山岳阙"、"内宫天号普济会"字样，中部钤朱印并书"驱邪降福"，下部书"镇宅平安"、阴阳八卦图及五岳名称和符号等。保存基本完好，纸张泛黄。

中华医学会 / 上海中医药大学医史博物馆藏

Used for counteracting evil force, the woodcutting figure was printed on the white paper and has been mounted with frame. In the upper part of the figure are some characters saying "the magic figure was made in Fahua Mountain", and the seal mark in middle part shows that the figure could counteract evil force and bring good luck. Yin and yang, the Eight Diagrams, Five Mountains and "Zhen Zhai Ping An" (stabilizing and protecting house) were engraved on the lower part. The magic figure is still in good condition with yellow discoloration.
Preserved in Chinese Medical Association/Museum of Chinese Medicine, Shanghai University of Traditional Chinese Medicine

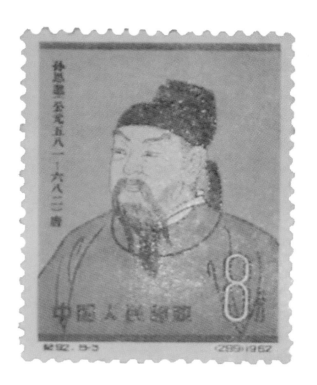
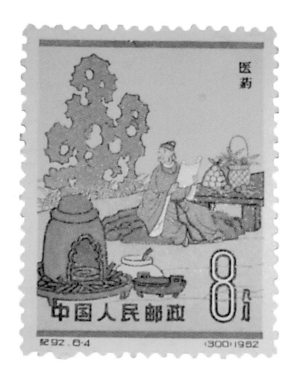

中国古代科学家邮票

近现代（1962）

长 3.6 厘米，宽 2.65 厘米，P111/2

Stamp of Ancient Chinese Scientist

Modern Times (1962)

Length 3.6 cm/ Width 2.65 cm/ P 111/2

Stamp Number "Ji 92.8-3"/Face Value 8 cents

长方形，为特种邮票。此票编号为"纪 92.8-3"，面值 8 分，是纪念隋唐著名医学家、药物学家孙思邈的两枚邮票。孙思邈，京兆华原（今陕西铜川市耀州区）人，医术高明，在针灸、疑难病症方面颇有成就，他总结前人和亲身经验，撰有《千金药方》《千金翼方》两部不朽医著。直形票，票面完好。1965 年入藏。

中华医学会 / 上海中医药大学医史博物馆藏

This vertical rectangular special stamp was issued to commemorate Sun Simiao, a famous medical scientist and pharmacologist in the Sui and Tang dynasties. Sun Simiao, from Huayuan in Jingzhao (now as Yaozhou District, Tongchuan City in Shaanxi Province), made great achievements in acupuncture and the treatment of difficult and complicated diseases. On the basis of the past and his own experiences, he created two immortal medical masterpieces *Qian Jin Yao Fang* (Thousand-Gold Prescriptions for Ready Use) and *Qian Jin Yi Fang* (Supplementary Prescriptions). The stamp was collected in 1965 and is still in good condition.

Preserved in Chinese Medical Association/Museum of Chinese Medicine, Shanghai University of Traditional Chinese Medicine

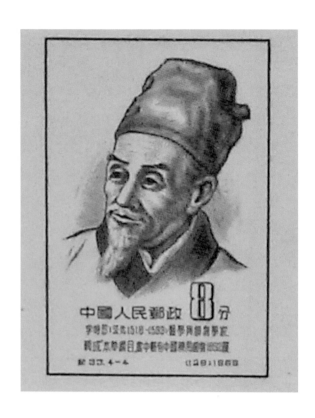

中国古代科学家（第一组）李时珍纪念邮票

近现代（1956）

长 9 厘米，宽 6.3 厘米，图案面积：2.7 厘米 ×4.3 厘米

编号"纪 33.4–4"，票面值为 8 分

Stamps of Ancient Chinese Scientists: Li Shizhen Commemorative Stamp

Modern Times (1956)

Length 9 cm/ Width 6.3 cm/ Picture Size 2.7 cm×4.3 cm

Stamp Number "Ji 33.4-4"/ Face Value 8 cents

长方形，为纪念邮票。全套"中国古代科学家（第一组）小型张"共四枚，画面分别是张衡、僧一行、李时珍和祖冲之像及各自取得的主要成就。此枚邮票画面为李时珍像。直形票，小型张，票面完好。1956 年入藏。

中华医学会 / 上海中医药大学医史博物馆藏

This vertical rectangular special stamp is the first small-sized one of the set of Stamps of Ancient Chinese Scientist, which records the figures of Zhang Heng, Seng Yixing, Li Shizhen and Zu Chongzhi as well as their main achievements. This stamp of Li Shizhen is still in good condition. It was collected in 1965.
Preserved in Chinese Medical Association/ Museum of Chinese Medicine, Shanghai University of Traditional Chinese Medicine

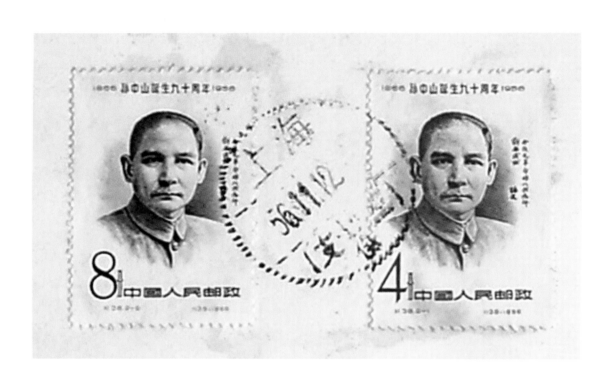

孙中山诞辰 90 周年纪念邮票

近现代（1956）

长 3.4 厘米，宽 2.2 厘米，P14

编号为"纪 38"，票面值为 4 分和 8 分

Commemorative Stamps for 90th Birthday of Sun Yat-sen

Modern Times (1956)

Length 3.4 cm/ Width 2.2 cm/ P 14

Stamp Number "Ji 38"/ Face Value 4 cents/ 8 cents

长方形，为纪念邮票。该套邮票一套两枚，专为纪念孙中山先生诞辰 90 周年发行。邮票上有孙中山像及"今后之革命非以俄为师断无成就"之题词。直形票，票面完好，盖点线边戳，戳上有"上海 56•11•12"字样，戳面较清晰。邮票粘贴于纸上。1958 年入藏。

中华医学会 / 上海中医药大学医史博物馆藏

Including two vertical rectangular stamps, this set of commemorative stamps was issued to commemorate the 90th birthday of Sun Yat-sen. On the stamps are Sun's head portrait and inscription written by him saying that "Chinese revolution must rely on the guidance of Russia". Stuck to the paper, the stamps are sealed with point-line postmark, which clearly reads the scripts of "Shanghai 56.11.12". This set of stamps was collected in 1958 and is still in good condition.

Preserved in Chinese Medical Association/ Museum of Chinese Medicine, Shanghai University of Traditional Chinese Medicine

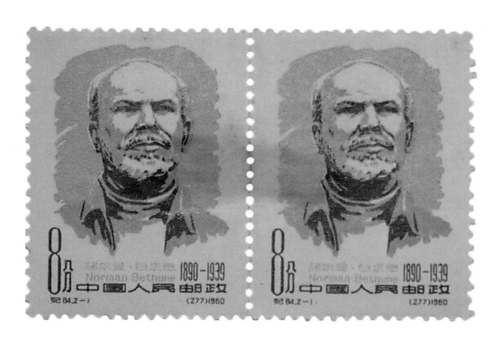

白求恩大夫像纪念邮票

近现代

长 3.4 厘米，宽 2.4 厘米，P11 1/2 × 11

编号为"纪 84.2-1"，票面值为 8 分

Commemorative Stamps for Doctor Bethune

Modern Times

Length 3.4 cm/ Width 2.4 cm/ P11 1/2 × 11

Stamp Number "Ji 84.2-1"/ Face Value 8 cents

长方形，为纪念邮票。该票于 1960 年（白
求恩诞辰 70 周年）11 月 20 日发行。直形票，
横双连，票面完整，略有褪色，背面有浆糊
粘贴粉红色纸张残迹，正面可见到粉红色浆
液浸渍。1960 年入藏。

中华医学会 / 上海中医药大学医史博物馆藏

These two vertical rectangular stamps in
horizontal pairs were issued to commemorate
the 70th birthday of Doctor Bethune on
November 20th, 1960. This set of stamps is in
good condition with little color fading. The pink
broken back paper and paste stain could still be
seen.

Preserved in Chinese Medical Association/
Museum of Chinese Medicine, Shanghai
University of Traditional Chinese Medicine

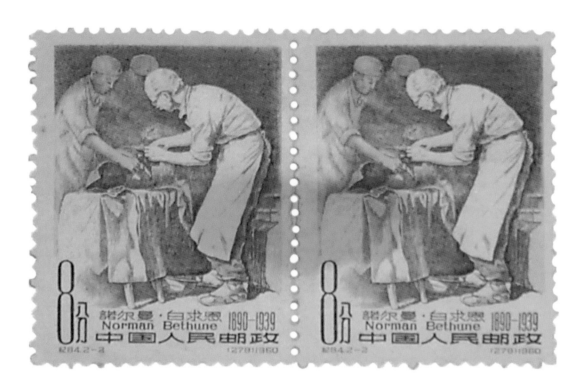

白求恩大夫在抢救伤员邮票

近现代

长 3.4 厘米，宽 2.4 厘米，P11 1/2 ×11

编号为"纪 84.2-1"，票面值为 8 分

Commemorative Stamps of Doctor Bethune Treating the Wounded

Modern Times

Length 3.4 cm/ Width 2.4 cm/ P11 1/2 × 11

Stamp Number "Ji 84.2-1"/ Face Value 8 cents

长方形，为纪念邮票。该票于 1960 年（白
求恩诞辰 70 周年）11 月 20 日发行。直形票，
横双连，票面完整，略有褪色，背面有浆糊
粘贴粉红色纸张残迹，正面可见到粉红色浆
液浸渍。1960 年入藏。

中华医学会 / 上海中医药大学医史博物馆藏

These two vertical rectangular stamps in
horizontal pairs were issued to commemorate
the 70th birthday of Doctor Bethune on
November 20th, 1960. This set of stamps is in
good condition with little color fading. The
pink broken back paper and paste stain could
still be seen.

Preserved in Chinese Medical Association/
Museum of Chinese Medicine, Shanghai
University of Traditional Chinese Medicine

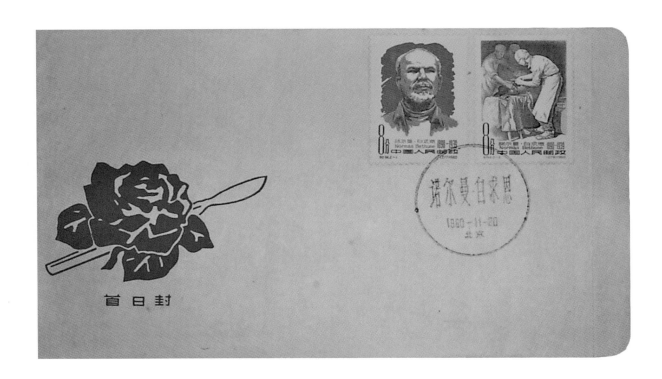

白求恩纪念首日封

近现代

16.6 厘米 ×10.2 厘米

编号为"纪 84.2–1"和"纪 84.2–2"，票面值为 8 分

Commemorative First-day Cover for Doctor Bethune

Modern Times

16.6 cm×10.2 cm

Stamp Number "Ji 84.2-1" "Ji 84.2-2"/ Face Value 8 cents

纪念封，为医事纪念品。该藏是为纪念白求恩诞辰 70 周年而发行的首日封。信封正面印有手术刀和牡丹花图样，右上角粘两枚白求恩纪念邮票为白求恩肖像；另枚为白求恩在前线为伤员做手术的图案。保存基本完好。1960 年入藏。

中华医学会 / 上海中医药大学医史博物馆藏

This first-day cover, a medical souvenir was issued to commemorate the 70th birthday of Doctor Bethune. On the front of the envelop are peony and scalpel and in the right upper corner are two commemorative stamps for doctor Bethune, among which is Bethune's portrait, and another is about Bethune operating on the wounded soldier. This first-day cover was collected in 1960 and is still in good condition. Preserved in Chinese Medical Association/ Museum of Chinese Medicine, Shanghai University of Traditional Chinese Medicine

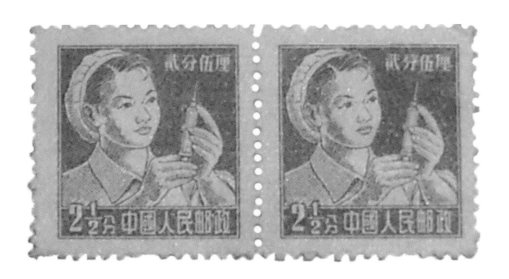

工农兵图案（医务工作者）普通邮票

近现代

长 2 厘米，宽 1.8 厘米，P14

编号为"普 8.9–4"，票面值为 2.5 分

Stamps of Worker-Peasant-Soldier (Medical Staff)

Modern Times

Length 2 cm/ Width 1.8 cm/ P14

Stamp Number "Pu 8.9-4"/ Face Value 2.5 cents

长方形，为普通邮票。该邮票为孔雀兰。"普8"
邮票，1955 年 7 月 16 日至 1956 年 12 月
25 日发行。全套邮票共 9 枚，均为工农兵图
案，依次为矿工、机械工人、空军战士、医
务工作者、陆军战士、冶金工人、科学工作
者、农妇、海军战士。胶版。横双连，直形票，
边白不匀称。1960 年入藏。

中华医学会 / 上海中医药大学医史博物馆藏

This set of stamps of worker-peasant-soldier,
with color of peacock orchid, was issued
during the period between July 16th, 1955 and
December 25th, 1956, including 9 stamps,
which were painted with miner, machinist,
airman, medical worker, soldier, metal worker,
scientist, peasant, and navy man respectively.
These vertical offset printing stamps of medical
workers are in horizontal pairs with the margin
color not evenly white. They were collected in
1960.

Preserved in Chinese Medical Association/
Museum of Chinese Medicine, Shanghai
University of Traditional Chinese Medicine

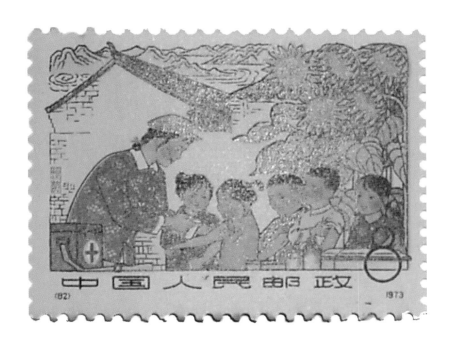

赤脚医生邮票

近现代

长 4 厘米，宽 3 厘米， P111/2 ×P11

Barefoot Doctor Stamp (82)

Modern Times

Length 4 cm/ Width 3 cm/ P111/2×P11

长方形，为普通邮票。画面为赤脚医生在预防接种。横行票，个别齿孔不规整。1974 年入藏。

中华医学会 / 上海中医药大学医史博物馆藏

The rectangular normal stamp shows that a barefoot doctor is vaccinating the children. The stamp is in the shape of horizontal rectangle with several irregular perforations. It was collected in 1974.

Preserved in Chinese Medical Association/ Museum of Chinese Medicine, Shanghai University of Traditional Chinese Medicine

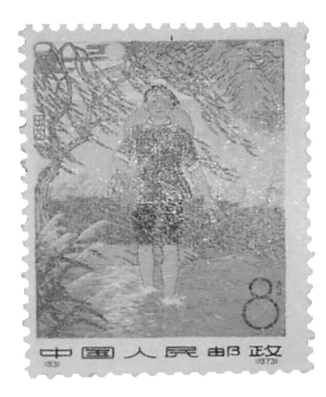

赤脚医生邮票

近现代

长 4 厘米，宽 3 厘米， P111/2 ×P11

长方形，为普通邮票。画面为赤脚医生出诊。直形票，个别齿孔不规整。1974 年入藏。

中华医学会 / 上海中医药大学医史博物馆藏

Barefoot Doctor Stamp (83)

Modern Times

Length 4 cm/ Width 3 cm/ P111/2×P11

The rectangular normal stamp shows that a barefoot doctor is visiting a patient at home. The stamp is in the shape of vertical rectangle with several irregular perforations. It was collected in 1974.

Preserved in Chinese Medical Association/Museum of Chinese Medicine, Shanghai University of Traditional Chinese Medicine

赤脚医生邮票

近现代

长 4 厘米，宽 3 厘米， P111/2 ×P11

长方形，为普通邮票。画面为赤脚医生在山间采
药。直形票，个别齿孔不规整。1974 年入藏。

中华医学会 / 上海中医药大学医史博物馆藏

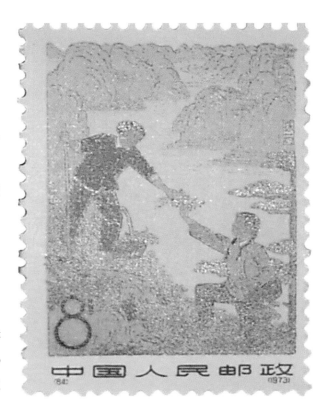

Barefoot Doctor Stamp (84)

Modern Times

Length 4 cm/ Width 3 cm/ P111/2×P11

The rectangular normal stamp shows that a barefoot
doctor is picking herbs in the mountains. The stamp
is in the shape of vertical rectangle with several
irregular perforations. It was collected in 1974.

Preserved in Chinese Medical Association/Museum
of Chinese Medicine, Shanghai University of
Traditional Chinese Medicine

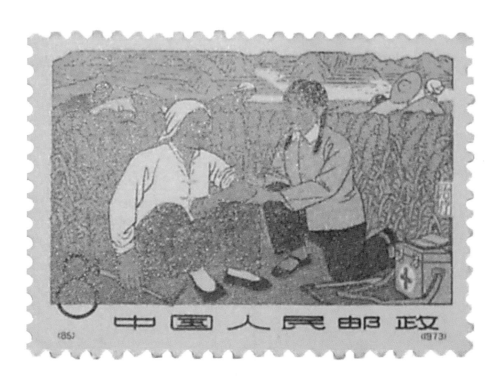

赤脚医生邮票

近现代

纸质

长 4 厘米，宽 3 厘米，P11×P111/2

Barefoot Doctor Stamp (85)

Modern Times

Length 4 cm/ Width 3 cm/ P11×P111/2

长方形，为普通邮票。此邮票标号为"编85"，是中华人民共和国成立后发行的文教卫生邮票之一，为编号邮票，面值8分，画面为赤脚医生在田间为农民治疗。赤脚医生是"文革"中对农村不脱产的基层卫生人员的称呼。这套邮票就是为纪念赤脚医生工作成绩所发行的邮票。横行票，个别齿孔不规整。1974年入藏。

中华医学会/上海中医药大学医史博物馆藏

The rectangular normal stamp labeled "No. 85" is one of the stamps of culture, education and hygiene published after the foundation of PRC. The face value of this labeled stamp is eight cents. It shows that a barefoot doctor is curing farmers in the field. Barefoot doctor is the name of the local health personnels who still keep their regular work in the Cultural Revolution period. The publishment of this set of stamps is to commemorate the barefoot doctors' contribution. The stamp is in the shape of horizontal rectangle with several irregular perforations. It was collected in 1974. Preserved in Chinese Medical Association/Museum of Chinese Medicine, Shanghai University of Traditional Chinese Medicine

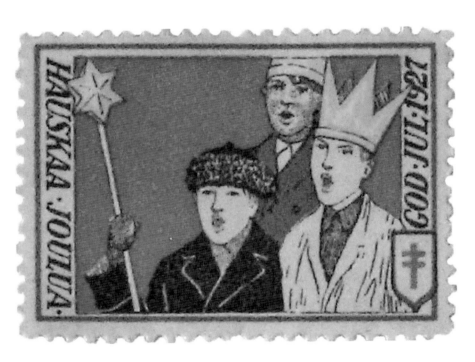

中国联合防痨邮票

近现代

长 4 厘米，宽 3 厘米

China United Anti-tuberculosis Stamp

Modern Times

Length 4 cm/ Width 3 cm

长方形，为邮票。该邮票为国际防痨邮票，票面为 3 个不同肤色的年青人做防痨宣传的场面。国际防痨协会成立于 20 世纪初，1902 年第一届国际防痨会议确定的标志为红双十字。美国 1912 年将双十字两端平头修改为 45° 宝剑式，取其含义是以武士精神杀魔鬼。它被称为美式双十字。这枚邮票上的标志为最初标志样式。横长连，基本完好，部分孔破损。1957 年入藏。

中华医学会 / 上海中医药大学医史博物馆藏

The rectangular international anti-tuberculosis stamp shows on the cover that three young people in different skin colors are doing anti-tuberculosis advertising. The IUATLD (The International Union Against Tuberculosis and Lung Disease) was founded in the beginning of 20th century. The first International Conference on Anti-tuberculosis in 1912 decided that the logo of it was red double cross. In 1912, America changed the two blunt ends of the double cross into sword-shaped ends in 45° with the meaning of killing the devils with the samurai spirit. The new double cross was also called American double cross. This stamp has the original logo. The basically intact stamps are linked horizontally with part of the perforations damaged. It was collected in 1957.

Preserved in Chinese Medical Association/Museum of Chinese Medicine, Shanghai University of Traditional Chinese Medicine

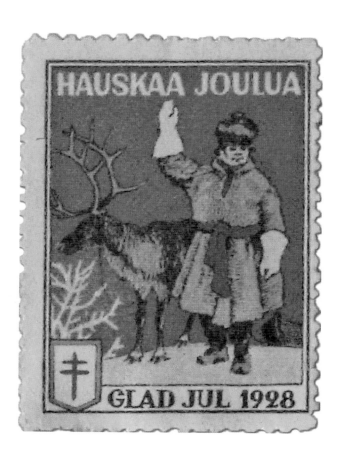

防痨纪念票

近现代

长 2.7 厘米，宽 2.1 厘米

The Commemorative Stamp of Anti-tuberculosis

Modern Times

Length 2.7 cm/ Width 2.1 cm

长方形，为邮票。该藏为国际防痨邮票式贺
年纪念票，票面为冬季里的一个牧人和一只
梅花鹿，画面有"HAUSKAA JOULUA"等
字样及美国防痨标志。直长连，基本完好，
部分孔破损。1957 年入藏。

中华医学会 / 上海中医药大学医史博物馆藏

The rectangular stamp is a New Year
commemorative stamp of international anti-
tuberculosis stamps. The cover of it shows
a shepherd and a sika deer with the words
of "HAUSKAA JOULUA" and the logo of
American anti-tuberculosis on it. This vertical
stamp is basically intact with part of the
perforations damaged. It was collected in 1957.
Preserved in Chinese Medical Association/
Museum of Chinese Medicine, Shanghai
University of Traditional Chinese Medicine

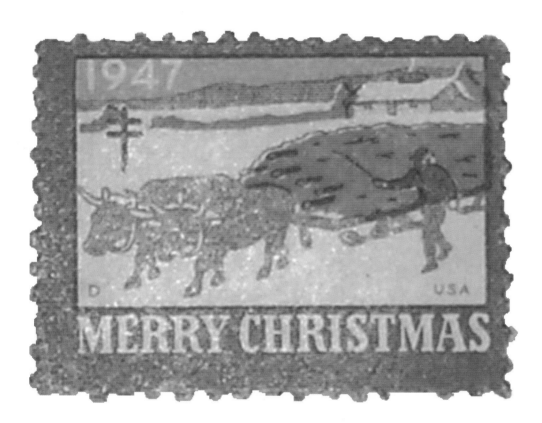

防痨纪念票

近现代

长 2.7 厘米，宽 2.1 厘米

The Commemorative Stamp of Anti-tuberculosis

Modern Times

Length 2.7 cm/ Width 2.1 cm

长 方 形，为 邮 票。该 藏 为 美 国 防 痨 邮 票
式 贺 年 纪 念 票，票 面 为 一 个 农 夫 赶 一 装
满 蔬 菜 的 牛 爬 犁，下 面 写 有 "MERRY
CHRISTMAS" 和 "USA" 等 字 样 及 美 国 防
痨 标 志。横 长 连，基 本 完 好，部 分 孔 破 损。
1961 年 入 藏。

中华医学会 / 上海中医药大学医史博物馆藏

The rectangular stamp is a New Year
commemorative stamp of America anti-
tuberculosis stamps. The cover of it shows
that a farmer is driving a cattle sledge full
of vegetables. At the bottom are the words
"MERRY CHRISTMAS", "USA" as well as the
America anti-tuberculosis logo. This horizontal
stamp is basically intact with part of the
perforations damaged. It was collected in 1961.
Preserved in Chinese Medical Association/
Museum of Chinese Medicine, Shanghai
University of Traditional Chinese Medicine

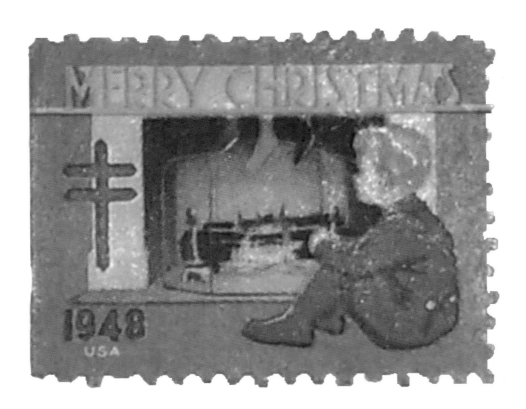

防痨纪念票

近现代

长 2.7 厘米，宽 2.1 厘米

The Commemorative Stamp of Anti-tuberculosis

Modern Times

Length 2.7 cm/ Width 2.1 cm

长方形，为邮票。该藏为美国防痨邮票式贺年纪念票，票面为一个儿童坐在壁炉旁，有"MERRY CHRISTMAS"和"USA"等字样及美国防痨标志。横长连，基本完好，部分孔破损。1961年入藏。

中华医学会 / 上海中医药大学医史博物馆藏

The rectangular stamp is a New Year commemorative stamp of America anti-tuberculosis stamps. The cover of it shows that a child is sitting beside a stove. There are the words "MERRY CHRISTMAS", "USA" as well as the America anti-tuberculosis logo on it. This horizontal stamp is basically intact with part of the perforations damaged. It was collected in 1961.

Preserved in Chinese Medical Association/ Museum of Chinese Medicine, Shanghai University of Traditional Chinese Medicine

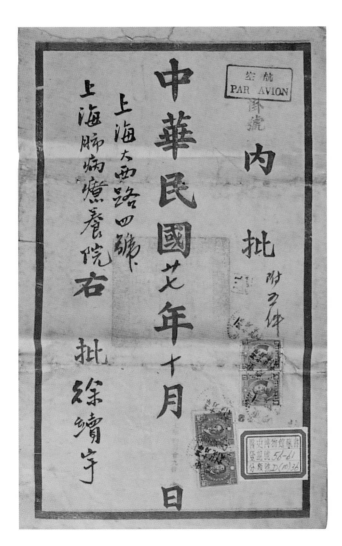

内政部卫生署封

近现代

32 厘米 ×18 厘米

The Envelop of the Department of
Health of Interior Ministry

Modern Times

32 cm×18 cm

信封，用于邮递。该藏为民国内政部卫生署邮寄函件的专门信封。正面除印有日期外，还填有"上海大西路四号上海市肺病疗养院徐续宇"字样，并粘邮票四枚，面值计6角8分，钤重庆发出邮局骑缝戳，上端钤有挂号航空印记。背面骑缝押内政部卫生署印章和到达局上海邮戳。保存基本完好。1956年入藏。

中华医学会／上海中医药大学医史博物馆藏

The envelop for mailing is the specialized envelop of Department of Health of Interior Ministry in Republican Period. Besides the date, the front of the envelope is also printed with "No. 4, Da Xi Road, Shanghai, Shanghai Lung Disease Sanatorium, Xu Xuyu (the address and the recipient) ". Four stamps with a total value of 68 cents are pasted on it. The stamp on the perforation is made by the sending post office in Chongqing. On the top is the imprint of registered airmail. The seal of Department of Health of Interior Ministry is on the perforation of the back as well as the seal of the receiving post office in Shanghai. It remains basically complete and was collected in 1956.

Preserved in Chinese Medical Association/Museum of Chinese Medicine, Shanghai University of Traditional Chinese Medicine

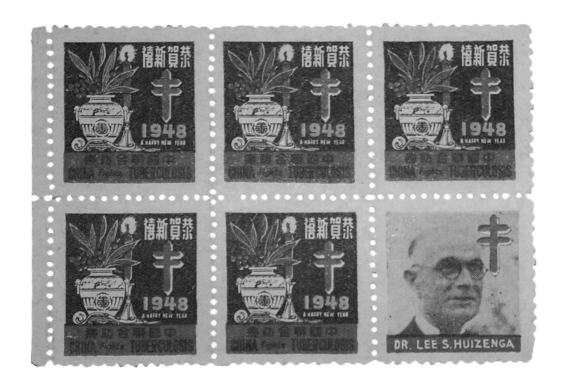

中国联合防痨邮票

近现代

长 2.8 厘米，宽 2.6 厘米，P11

China United Anti-tuberculosis Stamp

Modern Times

Length 2.8 cm/ Width 2.6 cm/ P11

长方形，为邮票。这套邮票是我国 1948 年 7 月发行的资助防痨附捐邮票，一共六枚，分两行相连，五枚相同图案，画面蓝、红两种底色，主图是花瓶和插花，另有"恭贺新禧"、"1948"、"中国联合防痨"、"CHINA Fights TUBERCULOSIS"字样及防痨标记；另一枚画面为 DR.LEE S.HUIZENGA 肖像。中国防痨协会 1933 年 11 月 21 日在上海成立时使用美式双十字标志，1948 年修改为两横线两端稍向上弯曲，象征我国独特的民族风格，中华人民共和国后继续沿用。直长连，基本完好，部分孔破损。1961 年入藏。

中华医学会 / 上海中医药大学医史博物馆藏

This set of rectangular stamps were issued in July, 1948, commemorating China to sponsor the anti-tuberculosis charity. The total six stamps are arranged and linked in two lines equally. Five of them are the same with blue and red background color and the main pattern of vase and flowers. Besides are the words "Gong He Xin Xi (Happy New Year)", "1948", "China United Anti-tuberculosis", "CHINA Fights TUBERCULOSIS" and the logo of anti-tuberculosis. Another one has the portrait of DR. LEE S. HUIZENGA on it. When Chinese Anti-tuberculosis Association was founded on November 21st, 1933 in Shanghai, the logo of American double cross was adopted. In 1948, the ends of two horizontal lines of the logo were changed into upward curved ends, representing the unique national style of China. It continued in use after 1949. The linked vertical stamps are basically intact with part of the perforations damaged. It was collected in 1961.

Preserved in Chinese Medical Association/Museum of Chinese Medicine, Shanghai University of Traditional Chinese Medicine

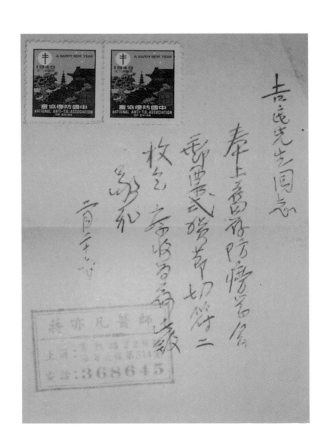

中国防痨协会邮票式贺年章

近现代

2.8 厘米 ×2.6 厘米

New Year Stamp of Chinese Anti-tuberculosis Association

Modern Times

2.8 cm ×2.6 cm

该藏用于纪念医事，是中国防痨协会于1949年新年之际发行的邮票式贺年章，一式两枚，粘于白纸上，是蒋亦凡医师赠给王吉民的贺节切符。保存基本完好。1961年入藏。

中华医学会 / 上海中医药大学医史博物馆藏

The New Year stamp is in memory of medical events, consisting of two pieces and was published by Chinese Anti-tuberculosis Associstion in the New Year of 1949, which is sticked on the white paper. It was the New Year card Doctor Jiang Yifan gave to Wang Jimin.The basically intact stamp was collected in 1961.

Preserved in Chinese Medical Association/ Museum of Chinese Medicine, Shanghai University of Traditional Chinese Medicine

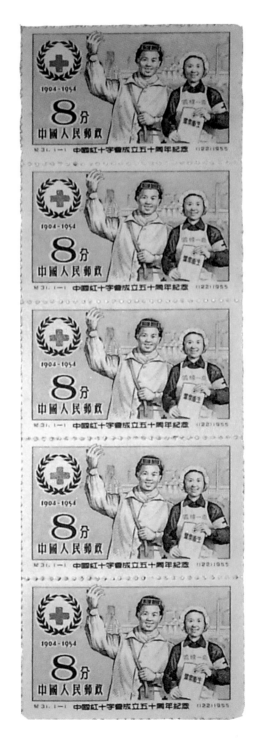

中国红十字会成立 50 周年纪念邮票

近现代

长 3.8 厘米，宽 2.2 厘米，P14

Commemorative Stamp of the 50th Anniversary of China Red Cross

Modern Times

Length 3.8 cm/ Width 2.2 cm/ P14

长方形，为纪念邮票。此邮票标号为"纪
31"，是新中国成立后发行的文教卫生纪念邮
票之一。中国红十字会成立于 1904 年，是我国
的人民卫生救护团体，主要从事组织红十字会员
积极开展卫生、献血、救护、护理、社会服务等
工作。横行票，五枚直长连，个别齿孔不规整。
1955 年入藏。

中华医学会 / 上海中医药大学医史博物馆藏

The number of the rectangular commemorative
stamp is "Ji 31". The stamp is one of the
commemorative stamps of culture, education and
hygiene issued after 1949. The Red Cross Society
of China was founded in 1904. It is a health rescue
organization of China and its members often
actively carry out the work such as hygiene, blood
donation, rescuing, nursing, social service and so
on. The stamp is in the shape of horizontal rectangle
with part of the perforations damaged. Every five
stamps are linked vertically. It was collected in
1955.

Preserved in Chinese Medical Association/Museum
of Chinese Medicine, Shanghai University of
Traditional Chinese Medicine

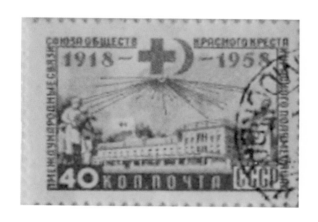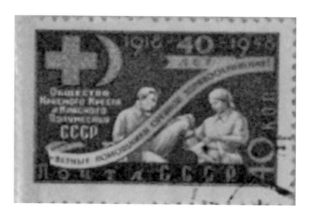

苏联红十字会红新月会联合会 40 周年纪念邮票

近现代

长 3.8 厘米，宽 2.6 厘米，P12

Commemorative Stamp of the 40th Anniversary of Red Cross and Red Crescent Societies

Modern Times

Length 3.8 cm/ Width 2.6 cm/ P12

长方形，为纪念邮票。两枚邮票上均有红"十"字
和"40"标记，其中一枚画面为前苏联红十字会大楼，
一枚为红十字会员在为患者服务的情形。红十字会
是一种志愿的、国际性的救护、救济团体。各国红
十字会的工作性质和范围等方面都有其独立性，在
苏联称红十字会与红新月会联合会。邮票为使用过
的旧票，有邮戳印记，但票面基本完好。1960年入藏。

中华医学会 / 上海中医药大学医史博物馆藏

The two rectangular commemorative stamps both have
a red cross and a number "40" on them. One of them
shows the mansion of Red Cross of the former Soviet
Union and the other shows that a member of Red Cross
is serving the patient. Red Cross is an international
volunteer organization of rescuing and relieving. The
Red Cross Society in every country is independent in
its work nature and serving range. In Soviet Union, it
was called the Soviet Union Federation of Red Cross
and Red Crescent Societies. Though the used stamp
has a postmark on it, its surface remains basically
undamaged. It was collected in 1960.

Preserved in Chinese Medical Association/Museum of
Chinese Medicine, Shanghai University of Traditional
Chinese Medicine

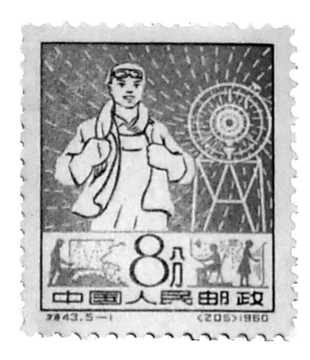

爱国卫生运动（厂矿卫生）特种邮票

近现代

长 2.6 厘米，宽 2.2 厘米，P111/2

长方形，为特种邮票。此票编号为"特 43.5 － 1"，以厂矿防暑降温为主题。直形票，票面完好。1960 年入藏。

中华医学会/上海中医药大学医史博物馆藏

The Special Stamp of the Patriotic Health Campaign (the Health of Factories and Mines)

Modern Times

Length 2.6 cm/ Width 2.2 cm/ P111/2

The rectangular special stamp is labeled "Te 43.5-1" and is themed of sunstroke prevention and lowering temperature of factories and mines. The stamp is in the shape of vertical rectangle and its surface remains basically undamaged. It was collected in 1960.

Preserved in Chinese Medical Association/Museum of Chinese Medicine, Shanghai University of Traditional Chinese Medicine

爱国卫生运动（讲卫生）特种邮票

近现代

长 2.6 厘米 , 宽 2.2 厘米，P111/2

长方形，为特种邮票。该藏编号为"特 43.5 – 3"，

以全民讲卫生爱清洁为主题。直形票，票面完好。

1960 年入藏。

中华医学会 / 上海中医药大学医史博物馆藏

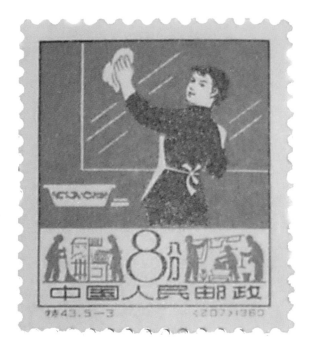

The Special Stamp of the Patriotic Health Campaign (Paying Attention to Hygiene)

Modern Times

Length 2.6 cm/ Width 2.2 cm/ P111/2

The rectangular special stamp is labeled "Te 43.5-3" and is themed of all the people paying attention to hygiene and often doing cleaning. The stamp is in the shape of vertical rectangle and its surface remains basically undamaged. It was collected in 1960.

Preserved in Chinese Medical Association/Museum of Chinese Medicine, Shanghai University of Traditional Chinese Medicine

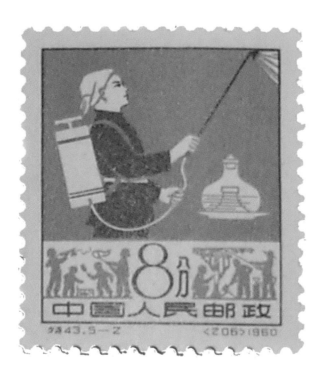

爱国卫生运动（除四害）特种邮票

近现代

长 2.6 厘米，宽 2.2 厘米

The Special Stamp of the Patriotic Health Campaign (Eliminating the Four Pests)

Modern Times

Length 2.6 cm/ Width 2.2 cm

长方形，为特种邮票。爱国卫生运动是毛泽东、周恩来 1952 年倡导的，是以除四害、讲卫生、消灭疾病为中心的群众卫生运动。为此邮电部于 1960 年 9 月 10 日发行"爱国卫生运动"特种邮票一套，共 5 枚，面值都是 8 分，包括厂矿卫生、除四害、讲卫生、预防疾病、锻炼身体五大主题。该藏编号为"特 43.5 – 2"，主图是农民在喷射杀虫药。直形票，票面完好。1960 年入藏。

中华医学会 / 上海中医药大学医史博物馆藏

The special stamp is rectangular. Advocated by Mao Zedong and Zhou Enlai in 1952, the Patriotic Health Campaign was a mass health campaign with five themes such as stressing on the health of factories and mines, eliminating the four pests, paying attention to hygiene, preventing diseases and exercising. This collection is labeled "Te 43.5-2". The main picture shows that a farmer is spraying insecticide. The stamp is in the shape of vertical rectangle and its surface remains basically undamaged. It was collected in 1960. Preserved in Chinese Medical Association/Museum of Chinese Medicine, Shanghai University of Traditional Chinese Medicine

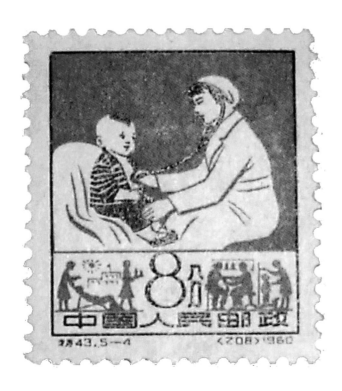

爱国卫生运动（预防疾病）特种邮票

近现代

长 2.6 厘米，宽 2.2 厘米，P111/2

The Special Stamp of the Patriotic Health Campaign (Preventing Diseases)

Modern Times

Length 2.6 cm/ Width 2.2 cm/ P111/2

长方形，为特种邮票。此票编号为"特
43.5－4"，以儿童健康检查预防疾病为主题。
直形票，票面完好。1960 年入藏。

中华医学会 / 上海中医药大学医史博物馆藏

The rectangular special stamp is labeled "Te
43.5-4" and is themed of children health
examination and disease prevention. The stamp
is in the shape of vertical rectangle and its
surface remains basically undamaged. It was
collected in 1960.

Preserved in Chinese Medical Association/
Museum of Chinese Medicine, Shanghai
University of Traditional Chinese Medicine

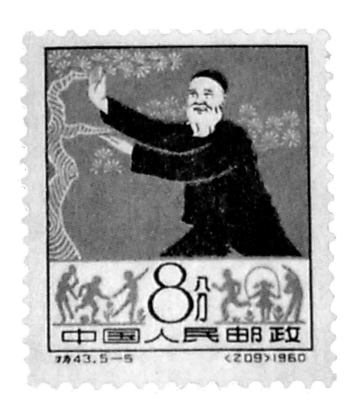

爱国卫生运动（锻炼身体）特种邮票

近现代

长 2.6 厘米，宽 2.2 厘米，P111/2

The Special Stamp of the Patriotic Health Campaign (Exercising)

Modern Times

Length 2.6 cm/ Width 2.2 cm/ P111/2

长方形，为特种邮票。该藏编号为"特43.5 – 5"，以老人打太极拳锻炼身体为主题。直形票，票面完好。1960 年入藏。

中华医学会 / 上海中医药大学医史博物馆藏

The rectangular special stamp labeled "Te 43.5-5" is about old people playing Tai Chi and exercising. The stamp is in the shape of vertical rectangle and its surface remains basically undamaged. It was collected in 1960.

Preserved in Chinese Medical Association/ Museum of Chinese Medicine, Shanghai University of Traditional Chinese Medicine

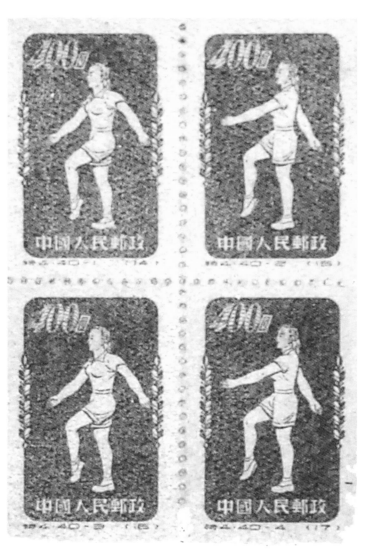

第一套广播体操邮票（第一节下肢运动）

近现代

长 6 厘米，宽 4 厘米，P121/2

单枚图案面积 2.55 厘米 ×1.6 厘米

The Stamp of the First Radio Calisthenics (The First Period: Legs Exercise)

Modern Times

Length 6 cm/ Width 4 cm/ P121/2

Size of Each Stamp 2.55 cm×1.6 cm

长 方 形，为 特 种 邮 票。此 邮 票 标 号 为 " 特 4.40 –
1/2/3/4"，红。1951 年 11 月 24 日公布了我国第一套成
人广播体操，并很快在全国范围开展锻炼。"特四"邮
票将第一套广播体操的十节动作，每节分为四个图案连
成一个方连，票面均为 400 元（人民币旧币值），全套
共 40 枚，形成完整的广播体操分解图。直行票，四方连，
有些齿孔不够清晰，相连邮票间齿孔纸屑几乎全未打落。
1960 年入藏。

中华医学会 / 上海中医药大学医史博物馆藏

The rectangular special stamp labeled "Te 4.40-1/2/3/4"
are red. On November 24th, 1951, the first Chinese radio
calisthenics for adults was published and soon spread all over
the China. The first radio calisthenics has ten periods and
in the set of "Special 4", and four patterns of every period
form a block. The face value of each stamp is 400 yuan (old
RMB value). The forty stamps of the whole set are complete
breakdown drawings of the radio calisthenics. The stamps
are in the shape of vertical rectangles and every four stamps
form a block. Some perforations are still not clear enough
and the perforations between the stamps are nearly all filled
with paper scraps. It was collected in 1960.
Preserved in Chinese Medical Association/Museum of
Chinese Medicine, Shanghai University of Traditional
Chinese Medicine

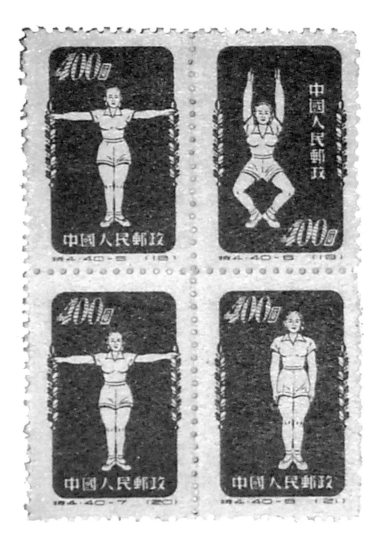

第一套广播体操邮票（第二节
四肢运动）

近现代

长 6 厘米，宽 4 厘米，P121/2

单枚图案面积 2.55 厘米 ×1.6 厘米

The Stamp of the First Radio Calisthenics (The Second Period: Exercise of the Four Limbs)

Modern Times

Length 6 cm/ Width 4 cm/ P121/2

Size of Each Stamp 2.55 cm× 1.6 cm

长方形，为特种邮票。此邮票标号为"特
4.40 – 37/38/39/40"，孔雀蓝。直行票，
四方连，齿孔不够清晰，孔内纸屑未打落。
1960 年入藏。

中华医学会 / 上海中医药大学医史博物馆藏

The rectangular special stamps are peacock blue
and are labeled "Te 4.40-37/38/39/40". The
stamps are in the shape of vertical rectangles
and every four stamps form a block. Some
perforations are still not clear enough and are
filled with paper scraps. It was collected in
1960.

Preserved in Chinese Medical Association/
Museum of Chinese Medicine, Shanghai
University of Traditional Chinese Medicine

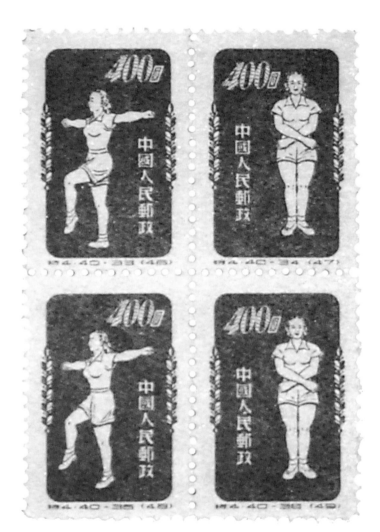

第一套广播体操邮票（第三节胸部运动）

近现代
长 6 厘米，宽 4 厘米，P121/2
单枚图案面积 2.55 厘米 ×1.6 厘米

The Stamp of the First Radio Calisthenics (The Third Period: Chest Exercise)

Modern Times
Length 6 cm/Width 4 cm/ P121/2
Size of Each Stamp 2.55 cm×1.6 cm

长方形，为特种邮票。此邮票标号为"特
4.40 – 9/10/11/12"，紫红。直行票，四方
连，齿孔不够清晰，邮票相连处齿孔纸屑全
未打落。1960 年入藏。

中华医学会 / 上海中医药大学医史博物馆藏

The rectangular special stamps are purplish
red and are labeled "Te 4.40-9/1011/12". The
stamps are in the shape of vertical rectangles
and every four stamps form a block. Some
perforations are still not clear enough and the
perforations between the stamps are nearly
all filled with paper scraps. It was collected in
1960.

Preserved in Chinese Medical Association/
Museum of Chinese Medicine, Shanghai
University of Traditional Chinese Medicine

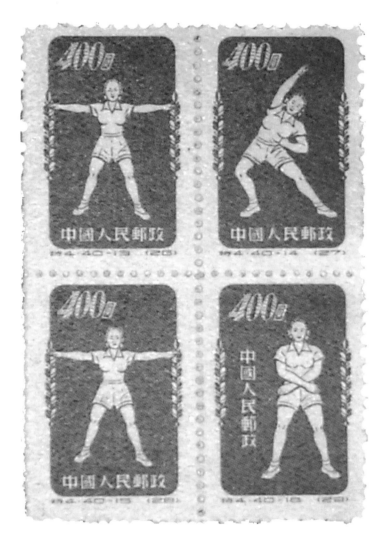

第一套广播体操邮票（第四节
体侧运动）

近现代
长 6 厘米，宽 4 厘米，P121/2
单枚图案面积 2.55 厘米 ×1.6 厘米

The Stamp of the First Radio Calisthenics (The Fourth Period: Side Exercise)

Modern Times
Length 6 cm/ Width 4 cm/ P121/2
Size of Each Stamp 2.55 cm×1.6 cm

长方形，为特种邮票。此邮票标号为"特
4.40 – 13/14/15/16"，草绿。直行票，四
方连，有些齿孔不够清晰，孔内纸屑未打落。
1960 年入藏。

中华医学会 / 上海中医药大学医史博物馆藏

The rectangular special stamps are grass green
and are labeled "Te 4.40-13/14/15/16". The
stamps are in the shape of vertical rectangles
and every four stamps form a block. Some
perforations are still not clear enough and are
filled with paper scraps. It was collected in
1960.

Preserved in Chinese Medical Association/
Museum of Chinese Medicine, Shanghai
University of Traditional Chinese Medicine

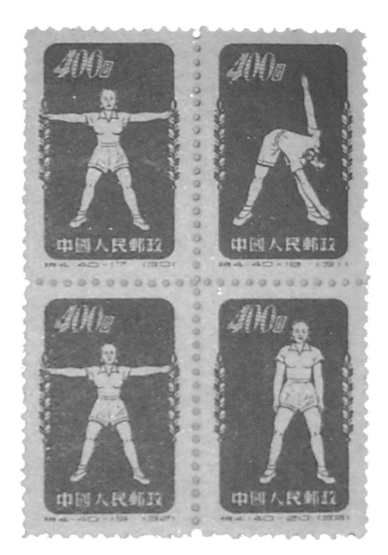

第一套广播体操邮票（第五节
转体运动）

近现代
长 6 厘米，宽 4 厘米，P121/2
单枚图案面积 2.55 厘米 ×1.6 厘米

**The Stamp of the First Radio
Calisthenics (The Fifth
Period: Twisting Exercise)**

Modern Times
Length 6 cm/ Width 4 cm/ P121/2
Size of Each Stamp 2.55 cm×1.6 cm

长方形，为特种邮票。此邮票标号为"特

4.40 – 17/18/19/20"，朱红。直行票，四方连，

齿孔清晰。1960 年入藏。

中华医学会 / 上海中医药大学医史博物馆藏

The rectangular special stamps are vermeil and
are labeled "Te 4.40-17/18/19/20". The stamps
are in the shape of vertical rectangles and every
four stamps form a block. Perforations are clear.
It was collected in 1960.
Preserved in Chinese Medical Association/
Museum of Chinese Medicine, Shanghai
University of Traditional Chinese Medicine

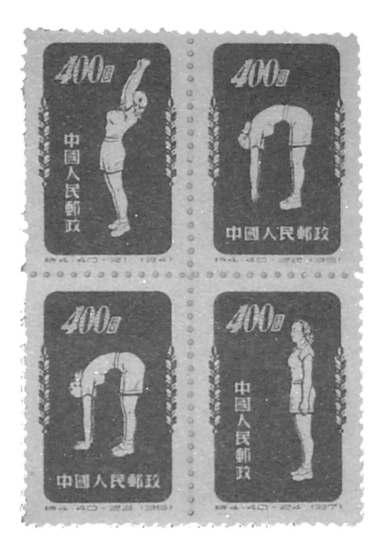

第一套广播体操邮票（第六节
腹背运动）

近现代
长 6 厘米，宽 4 厘米，P121/2
单枚图案面积 2.55 厘米 ×1.6 厘米

The Stamp of the First Radio Calisthenics (The Sixth Period: Exercise for Back and Belly)

Modern Times
Length 6 cm/ Width 4 cm/ P121/2
Size of Each Stamp 2.55 cm×1.6 cm

长方形，为特种邮票。此邮票标号为"特
4.40 – 21/22/23/24"，淡蓝。直行票，四方连，
个别齿孔纸屑未打落。1960 年入藏。

中华医学会 / 上海中医药大学医史博物馆藏

The rectangular special stamps are light blue
and are labeled "Te 4.40-21/22/23/24". The
stamps are in the shape of vertical rectangles
and every four stamps form a block. Some
perforations are still filled with paper scraps. It
was collected in 1960.
Preserved in Chinese Medical Association/
Museum of Chinese Medicine, Shanghai
University of Traditional Chinese Medicine

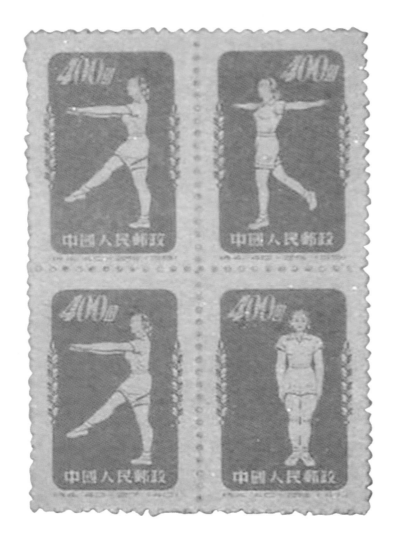

第一套广播体操邮票（第七节平衡运动）

近现代

长 6 厘米，宽 4 厘米，P121/2

单枚图案面积 2.55 厘米 ×1.6 厘米

The Stamp of the First Radio Calisthenics (The Seventh Period: Balancing Exercise)

Modern Times

Length 6 cm/ Width 4 cm/ P121/2

Size of Each Stamp 2.55 cm× 1.6 cm

长方形，为特种邮票。此邮票标号为"特 4.40 – 25/26/27/28"，桔黄。直行票，四方连，有些齿孔不够清晰，齿孔纸屑未打落。1960 年入藏。

中华医学会 / 上海中医药大学医史博物馆藏

The rectangular special stamps are orange and are labeled "Te 4.40-25/26/27/28". The stamps are in the shape of vertical rectangles and every four stamps form a block. Some perforations are still not clear enough and are filled with paper scraps. It was collected in 1960.

Preserved in Chinese Medical Association/ Museum of Chinese Medicine, Shanghai University of Traditional Chinese Medicine

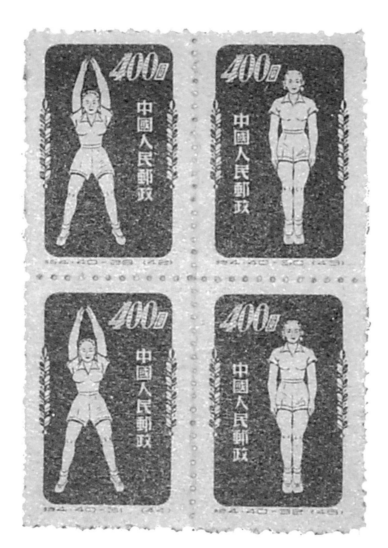

第一套广播体操邮票（第八节跳跃运动）

近现代
长 6 厘米，宽 4 厘米，P121/2
单枚图案面积 2.55 厘米 ×1.6 厘米

The Stamp of the First Radio Calisthenics (The Eighth Period: Jumping Exercise)

Modern Times
Length 6 cm/ Width 4 cm/ P121/2
Size of Each Stamp 2.55 cm×1.6 cm

长方形，为特种邮票。此邮票标号为"特
4.40 – 29/30/31/32"，深紫。直行票，四
方连，有些齿孔不够清晰，齿孔纸屑未打落。
1960 年入藏。

中华医学会 / 上海中医药大学医史博物馆藏

The rectangular special stamps are deep purple
and are labeled "Te 4.40-29/30/31/32". The
stamps are in the shape of vertical rectangles
and every four stamps form a block. Some
perforations are still not clear enough and are
filled with paper scraps. It was collected in
1960.

Preserved in Chinese Medical Association/
Museum of Chinese Medicine, Shanghai
University of Traditional Chinese Medicine

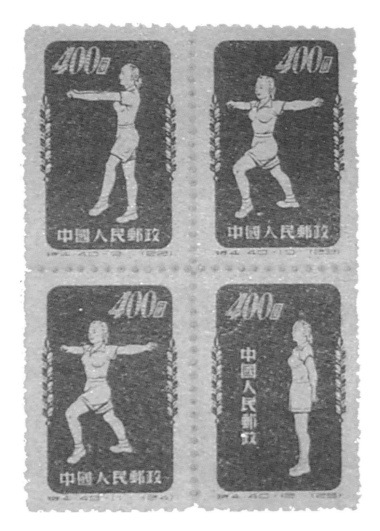

第一套广播体操邮票（第九节
整理运动）

近现代
长 6 厘米，宽 4 厘米，P121/2
单枚图案面积 2.55 厘米 ×1.6 厘米

The Stamp of the First Radio Calisthenics (The Ninth Period: Settling Exercise)

Modern Times
Length 6 cm/ Width 4 cm/ P121/2
Size of Each Stamp 2.55 cm× 1.6 cm

长方形，为特种邮票。此邮票标号为"特
4.40 – 33/34/35/36"，赭石。直行票，四
方连，有些齿孔不够清晰，齿孔纸屑未打落。
1960 年入藏。

中华医学会 / 上海中医药大学医史博物馆藏

The rectangular special stamps are ochre-
colored and are labeled "Te 4.40-33/34/35/36".
The stamps are in the shape of vertical
rectangles and every four stamps form a block.
Some perforations are still not clear enough and
are filled with paper scraps. It was collected in
1960.

Preserved in Chinese Medical Association/
Museum of Chinese Medicine, Shanghai
University of Traditional Chinese Medicine

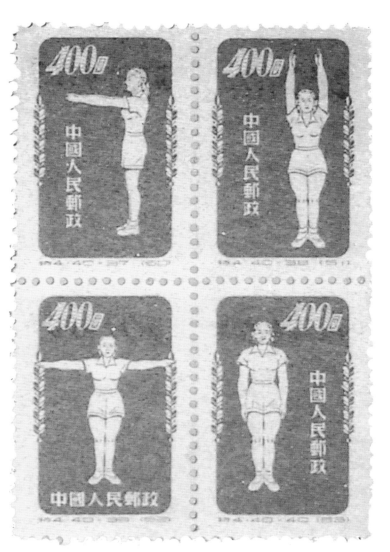

第一套广播体操邮票（第十节呼吸运动）

近现代
长 6 厘米，宽 4 厘米，P121/2
单枚图案面积 2.55 厘米 ×1.6 厘米

The Stamp of the First Radio Calisthenics (The Tenth Period: Breathing Exercise)

Modern Times
Length 6 cm/ Width 4 cm/ P121/2
Size of Each Stamp 2.55 cm× 1.6 cm

长方形，为特种邮票。此邮票标号为"特
4.40 – 37/38/39/40"，孔雀蓝。直行票，
四方连，个别齿孔不规整。1960 年入藏。

中华医学会 / 上海中医药大学医史博物馆藏

The rectangular special stamps are peacock blue
and are labeled "Te 4.40-37/38/39/40". The
stamps are in the shape of vertical rectangles
and every four stamps form a block. Some
perforations are not regular. It was collected in
1960.

Preserved in Chinese Medical Association/
Museum of Chinese Medicine, Shanghai
University of Traditional Chinese Medicine

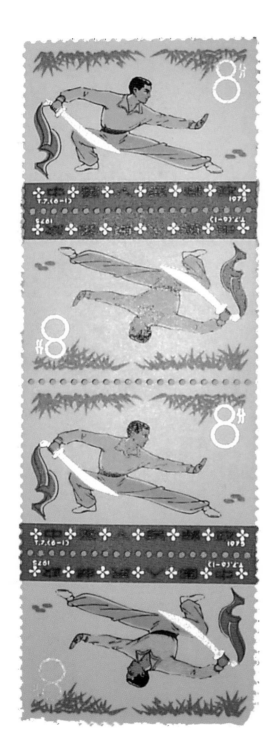

武术邮票

近现代

长 4 厘米，宽 3 厘米，P111/2 ×P11

The Stamp of Martial Arts

Modern Times

Length 4 cm/ Width 3 cm/ P111/2×P11

长方形，为特种邮票。此邮票标号为"T.7(1)"，是中华人民共和国成立后发行的体育运动邮票之一，为特种邮票，面值8分。该票画面为刀术，为对倒印刷票。武术在中国源远流长，有广泛的群众基础，是中华民族光辉灿烂文化遗产的一部分。这套邮票是为纪念毛泽东同志"发展体育运动，增强人民体质"题词发表23周年而发行的。横行票，个别齿孔不规整。1976年入藏。

中华医学会/上海中医药大学医史博物馆藏

The rectangular special stamp is labeled "T.7(1)". As one of the stamps of physical exercise issued after the foundation of PRC, this stamp is a special stamp with face value of eight cents. The stamp shows knife techniques. With a solid mass base, the long-standing and well-established martial arts have already become part of Chinese glorious cultural heritage. This set of stamps was issued in memory of the 23rd anniversary of Mao Zedong's inscription "Promote physical culture and build up the people's health". These tete-beche stamps are in the shape of horizontal rectangle with several irregular perforations. It was collected in 1976.

Preserved in Chinese Medical Association/Museum of Chinese Medicine, Shanghai University of Traditional Chinese Medicine

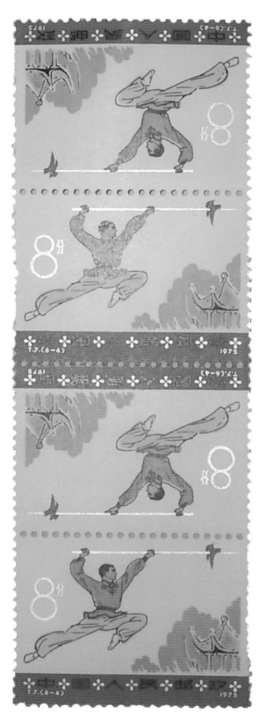

武术邮票

近现代

长 4 厘米，宽 3 厘米，P111/2 ×P11

长方形，为特种邮票。该票画面为枪术，为对倒印刷票。

横行票，个别齿孔不规整。1976 年入藏。

中华医学会 / 上海中医药大学医史博物馆藏

The Stamp of Martial Arts

Modern Times

Length 4 cm/ Width 3 cm/ P111/2×P11

The special stamp is rectangular. It shows spear techniques and was printed centrosymmetrically. The stamps are in the shape of horizontal rectangle with some irregular perforations. It was collected in 1976.

Preserved in Chinese Medical Association/Museum of Chinese Medicine, Shanghai University of Traditional Chinese Medicine

武术邮票

近现代

长 4 厘米，宽 3 厘米，P111/2 ×P11

长方形，为特种邮票。该票画面为剑术，为对倒印刷票。

横行票，个别齿孔不规整。1976 年入藏。

中华医学会 / 上海中医药大学医史博物馆藏

The Stamp of Martial Arts

Modern Times

Length 4 cm/ Width 3 cm/ P111/2×P11

The special stamp is rectangular. The stamp shows sword techniques. These tete-beche stamps are in the shape of horizontal rectangles with some irregular perforations. It was collected in 1976.

Preserved in Chinese Medical Association/Museum of Chinese Medicine, Shanghai University of Traditional Chinese Medicine

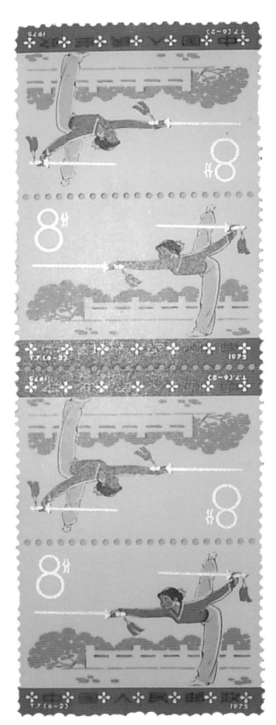

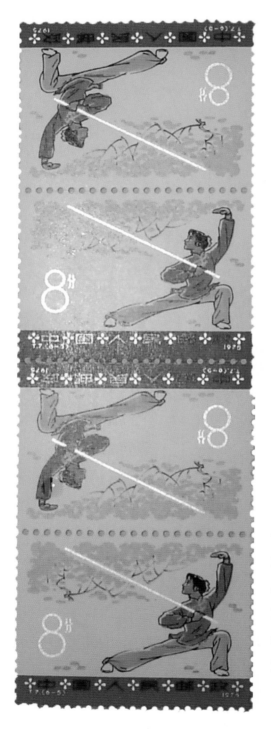

武术邮票

近现代

长4厘米，宽3厘米，P111/2 ×P11

长方形，为特种邮票。该票画面为棍术，为对倒印刷票。

横行票，个别齿孔不规整。1976年入藏。

中华医学会 / 上海中医药大学医史博物馆藏

The Stamp of Martial Arts

Modern Times

Length 4 cm/ Width 3 cm/ P111/2×P11

The special stamp is rectangular. The stamp shows cudgel techniques. These tete-beche stamps are in the shape of horizontal rectangles with some irregular perforations. It was collected in 1976.

Preserved in Chinese Medical Association/Museum of Chinese Medicine, Shanghai University of Traditional Chinese Medicine

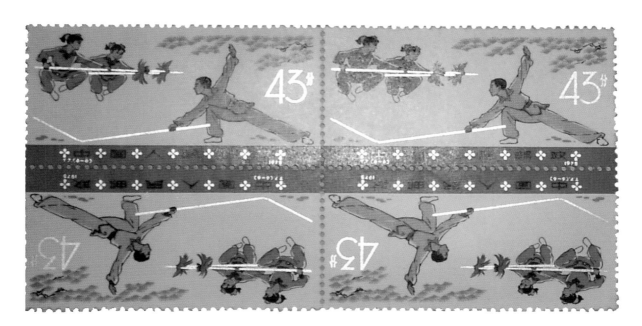

武术邮票

近现代

长 4 厘米　宽 3 厘米，P111/2 ×P11

长方形，为特种邮票。该票画面为三节棍对双枪，为对倒印刷票。横行票，个别齿孔不规整。1976 年入藏。

中华医学会 / 上海中医药大学医史博物馆藏

Martial Arts Stamp

Modern Times

Length 4 cm/ Width 3 cm/ P111/2 × P11

This is a special stamp in rectangular shape, showing a three-section cudgel against a double-edged spear on it.

These tete-beche stamps are horizontal with some irregular perforations. This stamp was collected in 1976.

Preserved in Chinese Medical Association/Museum of Chinese Medicine, Shanghai University of Traditional Chinese Medicine

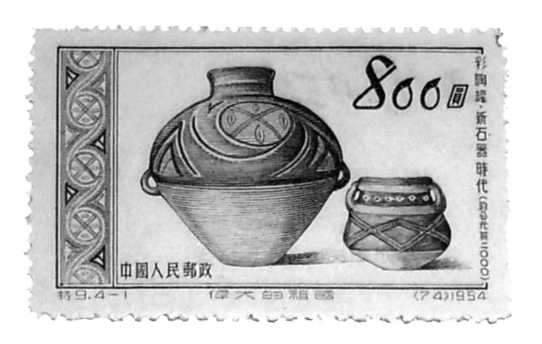

古代文物特种邮票（马厂类型彩陶瓮、罐）

近现代

长 3.65 厘米，宽 2.2 厘米，P14

Special Stamp of Ancient Cultural Relics (The Ancient Painted Pottery Jar and Pot of Machang Style)

Modern Times

Length 3.65 cm/ Width 2.2 cm/ P14

长方形，为特种邮票。此邮票标号为"特
9.4 - 1"，深棕。彩陶罐产生于新石器时期。
邮票上右边彩陶小罐纹样是双交叉折线纹，
左边彩陶瓮纹样是变幻的螺旋纹衬托下的大
圆圈纹，圆圈中还填以十字纹。横行票，票
面完好，但齿孔不规整。1960 年入藏。

中华医学会 / 上海中医药大学医史博物馆藏

This is a special stamp in rectangular shape and
dark brown color. The label of this stamp is "Te
9.4-1". The ancient painted pottery pots were
produced in the Neolithic Age. The painted
pottery pot is on the right side of the stamp,
with double crossed broken lines; on the left
is the painted pottery jar, with patterns of big
circles set off by changing spiral marks, and
there are also cross patterns inside those big
circles. This stamp was collected in 1960. It is a
transverse stamp with intact face and irregular
perforations.

Preserved in Chinese Medical Association/
Museum of Chinese Medicine, Shanghai
University of Traditional Chinese Medicine

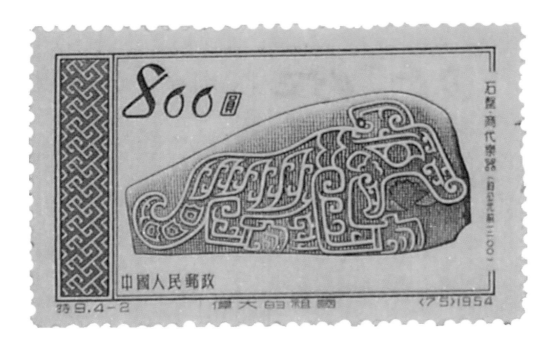

古代文物特种邮票（商代虎纹大石磬）

近现代

长 3.65 厘米，宽 2.2 厘米，P14

Special Stamp of Ancient Cultural Relic (Stone Chime with Tiger Pattern of Shang Dynasty)

Modern Times

Length 3.65 cm/ Width 2.2 cm/ P14

长方形，为特种邮票。此邮票标号为"特
9.4 － 2"，灰。票面上将"磬"误为"罄"，
该大石磬1950年春在河南安阳武官村商代
大墓出土。横行票，票面完好，但齿孔不规整。
1960年入藏

中华医学会/上海中医药大学医史博物馆藏

This is a special stamp in rectangular shape
and gray color, with the label "Te 9.4-2".
It mistakenly writes " 罄 "as " 磬 " on the
stamp. This stone chime was unearthed from
the large Shang tomb in Wuguan Village,
Anyang City, Henan Province, in the spring of
1950. This stamp was collected in 1960. It is a
transverse stamp with intact face and irregular
perforations.
Preserved in Chinese Medical Association/
Museum of Chinese Medicine, Shanghai
University of Traditional Chinese Medicine

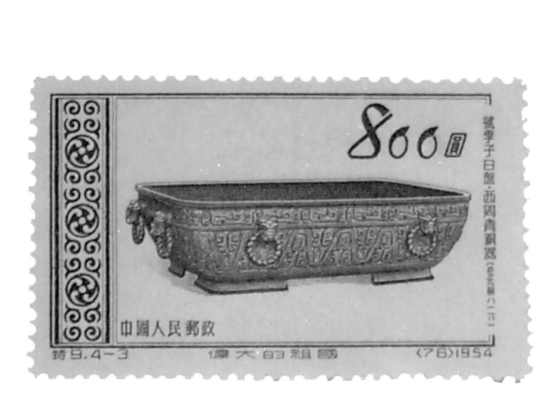

古代文物特种邮票（虢季子白盘）

近现代

长 3.65 厘米，宽 2.2 厘米，P14

Special Stamp of Ancient Cultural Relic (Ji Zibai Plate of the Guo State)

Modern Times

Length 3.65 cm/ width 2.2 cm/ P14

长方形，为特种邮票。此邮票标号为"特
9.4－3"，靛绿。盘是盥洗器，邮票上这
件长方形盘是传世最大的西周晚期铜器，于
周宣王十二年制作。横行票，票面完好，但
齿孔不规整。1960 年入藏。

中华医学会 / 上海中医药大学医史博物馆藏

This is a special stamp in rectangular shape and
indigo green color, with the label "Te 9.4-3". In
ancient times, the plate was used for washing
one's face and hands. This rectangular plate
on the stamp is the largest one of those bronze
wares of the late Western Zhou Dynasty that
have been handed down from ancient times, and
it was produced in the 12th year of the reign of
King Xuan of the Zhou Dynasty. This stamp
was collected in 1960. It is a transverse stamp
with intact face and irregular perforations.
Preserved in Chinese Medical Association/
Museum of Chinese Medicine, Shanghai
University of Traditional Chinese Medicine

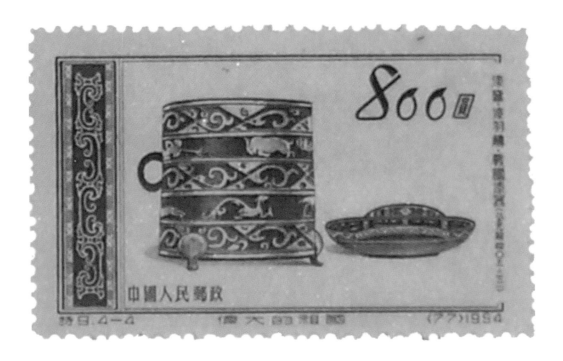

古代文物特种邮票（兽猎纹漆奁、漆羽觞）

近现代

长 3.65 厘米，宽 2.2 厘米，P14

Special Stamp of Ancient Cultural Relics (Lacquer Mirror Case with Hunting Pattern and Lacquer Wine Cup)

Modern Times

Length 3.65 cm/ Width 2.2 cm/ P14

长方形，为特种邮票。此邮票标号为"特9.4 – 4"，紫红。1952年
长沙颜家岭35号楚墓出土了一批战国时期漆器，邮票上的文物是其中
之一。大的是狩猎纹漆奁，是古代妇女梳妆用的镜盒；小的是羽觞，
即耳杯，是古代的酒杯。"特9"邮票全称"伟大的祖国（第五组）
古代文物特种邮票"，1954年8月25日发行，全套邮票共四枚，票
面均为800圆（人民币旧币值），画面为我国古代的几件珍贵文物。
横行票，票面完好，但齿孔不规整。1960年入藏。

中华医学会／上海中医药大学医史博物馆藏

This is a special stamp in rectangular shape and purplish red color, with the
label "Te 9.4-4". A batch of lacquer wares of the Warring States Period were
unearthed from No. 35 Chu Tomb at Yanjialing of Changsha City, Hunan
Province, and these two relics on the stamp are among them. The larger one
is the lacquer mirror case with hunting pattern, which was used by ancient
women for making up; the smaller one is the lacquer wine cup, also called
ear cup, used as the drinking vessel in ancient times. The full name of the
"Te 9" stamp series is "Special Stamp of Ancient Cultural Relic of Great
Motherland (The Fifth Set)". This set of stamp was issued on August 25,
1954, consisting of 4 stamps with the pictures of several precious cultural
relics of ancient China, and the par of each stamp is 800 Yuan (the old value
for RMB). This stamp was collected in 1960. It is a transverse stamp with
intact face and irregular perforations.

Preserved in Chinese Medical Association/Museum of Chinese Medicine,
Shanghai University of Traditional Chinese Medicine

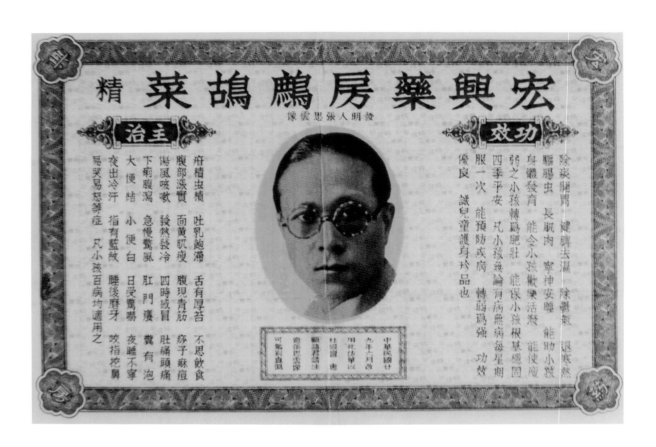

宏兴药房广告

近现代

长 18.5 厘米，宽 12.5 厘米

Advertisement of Hongxing Drugtore

Modern Times

Length 18.5 cm/ Width 12.5 cm

广东省潮州市宏兴药房鹧鸪菜广告。鹧鸪菜
主要分布于我国 广东、福建、浙江沿海，具
有驱虫杀虫、健脾化痰消积、安神之功效。

朱德明藏

This was an advertisement of Hongxing
Drugtore in Chaozhou City, Guangdong
Province, for caloglossa leprieurii. Mainly
distributed in coastal regions of China, like
Guangdong, Fujian and Zhejiang Province,
caloglossa leprieurii has effects of killing
ascaris lumbricoides, invigorating spleen,
removing phlegm, resolving food stagnancy and
tranquilizing.

Preserved by Zhu Deming

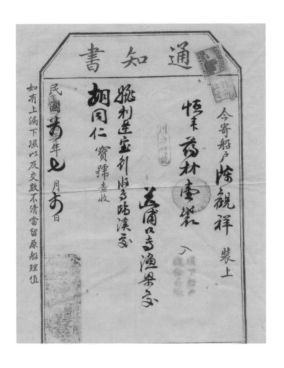

货单

近现代

长 30.5 厘米，宽 20.5 厘米

Bill of Lading (B/L)

Modern Times

Length 30.5 cm/ Width 20.5 cm

地处杭州望仙桥河下 23 号（砚瓦街口）恒
丰药行寄送的药材提货单。

朱德明藏

The bill of lading was delivered by Hengfeng
Drugstore located at No. 23 (Yanwa street)
under Wangxian Bridge of Hangzhou City.
Preserved by Zhu Deming

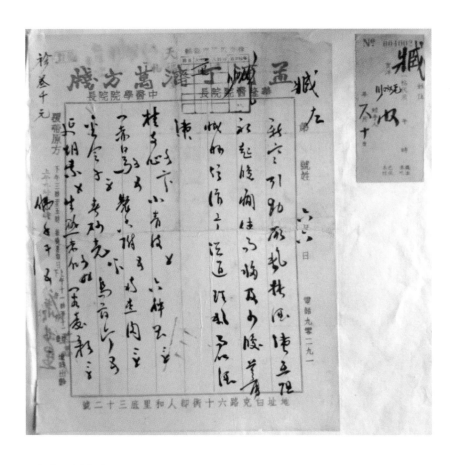

丁济万处方

近现代

长 27.5 厘米，宽 20.5 厘米

Prescription Written by Ding Jiwan

Modern Times

Length 27.5 cm/ Width 20.5 cm

丁济万〔1903—1963〕，丁甘仁之长孙，孟河丁氏医派的代表人物。他临证经验丰富，尤精内、外、妇、儿诸科，并热心于中医教育事业，曾任上海中医学院院长及上海国医学会理事长，并主持上海华隆中医院、南北广益善堂等机构，后移居香港及台湾行医。此为其在1946年6月6日上海市白克路60街〔即人和里底32号〕中医院手书处方。

朱德明藏

Ding Jiwan (1903-1963), the eldest grandson of Ding Ganren, was one of the representatives of the Ding's as a branch of Menghe Medical School. With rich clinical experience, Ding Jifang particularly specialized in internal medicine, surgery, gynecology and obstetrics, pediatrics and was very enthusiastic about Traditional Chinese Medicine education. Ding was once the president of Shanghai University of Traditional Chinese Medicine and the chairman of Shanghai Association of Traditional Chinese Medicine. He also chaired institutions like Shanghai Hualong Chinese Medicine Hospital, Southern and Northern Yishan Drugstore and so on. Afterwards, he moved to Hongkong and Taiwan working as a doctor. This prescription was written by him at Chinese Medicine Hospital in June 6th, 1946, which was previously located at the 60th Street, Baike Road, Shanghai City.

Preserved by Zhu Deming

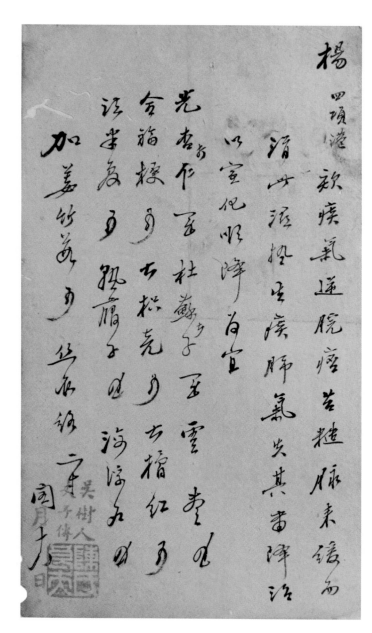

陈良夫处方

近现代

长 24 厘米，宽 13.5 厘米

Prescription Written by Chen Liangfu

Modern Times

Length 24 cm/ Width 13.5 cm

陈良夫 (1868—1920)，嘉善魏塘镇人。清光绪十三年 (1887) 中秀才，后弃儒习医，师事同县名医吴树人，精于切诊，长于时症，亦擅调理，对肝病更为擅长。行医 30 年，名盛当时。此为其手书处方。

朱德明藏

Chen Liangfu (1868-1920) was born in Weitang Town, Jiashan County. During the reign of Emperor Guangxu of Qing Dynasty, Chen became a Xiucai (a kind of distinguished talent topping at county level in ancient Chinese imperial examination), but later he chose to be a doctor instead of a scholar. As the student of a famous doctor from the same county called Wu Shuren, he was good at feeling the pulse, treating the epidemics, coordinating the body and curing liver diseases. He devoted himself to medicine for 30 years and gained great fame for a time. This is one prescription written by him.

Preserved by Zhu Deming

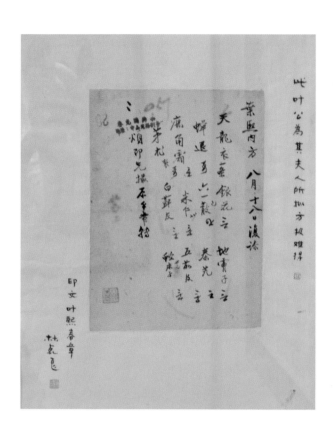

叶熙春处方

近现代

长 19 厘米，宽 13.5 厘米

Prescription written by Ye Xichun

Modern Times

Length 19 cm/ Width 13.5 cm

叶熙春早年师从杭州良渚名中医莫尚古，深得其旨。浙江名医姚梦兰延其侍诊 2 年，医术猛进。他精通内科、妇科，蜚声浙北。1929 年，赴上海行医，江、浙、皖诸省慕名求医者接踵。1946 年，与丰子恺、潘天寿等人发起恢复明远学社。此为 1949 年 8 月 18 日在家中为其夫人手书处方。

朱德明藏

Ye Xichun was early apprenticed to a renowned doctor, Mo Shanggu in Liangzhu Town, Hangzhou City, with good achievement. After two years of assistance to another renowned doctor Yao Menglan in Zhejiang Province, he got his expertise advanced dramatically. Since he specialized in internal medicine, gynecology and obstetrics, he gained fame and reputation in the north of Zhejiang Province. In 1929, Ye worked as a doctor in Shanghai and patients from Jiangxi, Zhejiang, Anhui and other provinces came to see him on purpose. In 1946, Feng Zikai, Pan Tianshou, Ye Xichun and others launched the resumption of Mingyuan Society. This prescription was written by Ye at home for his wife.

Preserved by Zhu Deming

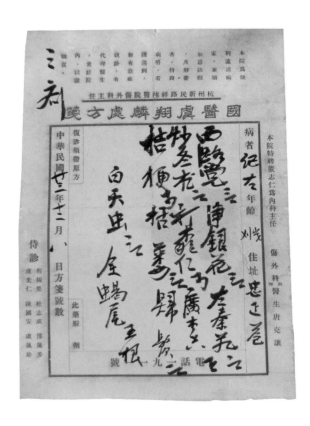

虞翔麟处方

近现代

长 31 厘米，宽 21.5 厘米

Prescription Written by Yu Xianglin

Modern Times

Length 31 cm/ Width 21.5 cm

虞翔麟是近代著名伤外科医师。1934 年 6 月 24 日，他倡导创立了近代中国第一所中医疗养院——西湖中医虚损疗养院，自任院长，聘请浙江省财政厅厅长王澂莹为名誉院长。此为 1934 年 12 月 8 日在杭州新民路祥林医院手书处方。

朱德明藏

Yu Xianglin was a renowned surgeon in Chinese modern times. On June 24th 1934, he advocated and established the first Chinese medicine sanatorium in modern times—West Lake Chinese Medicine Sanatorium. He appointed himself as the president of this sanatorium and also appointed the head of Zhejiang Provincial Department of Finance, Wang Chengying as the honorary president. This prescription was written by him in Xianglin hospital located on Xinmin Road, Zhejiang Province.

Preserved by Zhu Deming

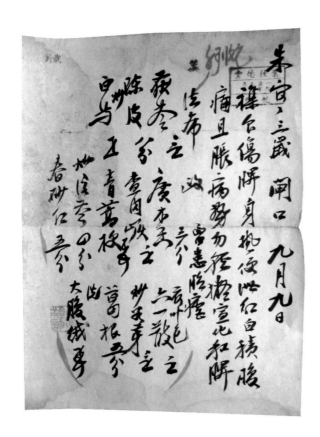

詹子翔处方

近现代

长 26 厘米，宽 18.5 厘米

Prescription Written by Ye Xichun

Modern Times

Length 26 cm/ Width 18.5 cm

詹子翔（1890—1954），出身于杭州市上城区丰乐桥小儿科世家，尤善医治小儿麻疹、疳积、泄泻、咳嗽等常见疾病，曾任杭州市中医院院长。此为 1920 年 9 月 9 日在杭州叶种德堂手书处方。

朱德明藏

Zhan Zixiang (1890-1954) was born in a family of pediatricians, under Fengle Bridge, Shangcheng District, Hangzhou City. He particularly specialized in treating common ailments like child-measles, infantile malnutrition, diarrhea, and cough. He once worked as the president of Hangzhou Hospital of Traditional Chinese Medicine. This prescription was written by him for Ye Zhongde Drugstore on September 9th, 1920.

Preserved by Zhu Deming

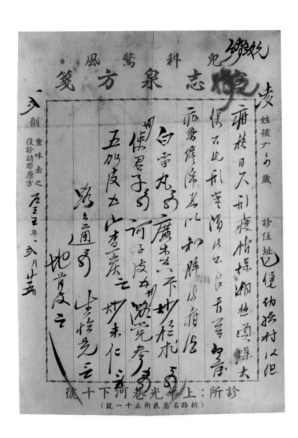

宣志泉处方

近现代

长 26.5 厘米，宽 17.5 厘米

Prescription Written by Yi Zhiquan

Modern Times

Length 26.5 cm/ Width 17.5 cm

宣志泉（1910—1977），杭州儿科名医，中华人民共和国成立初浙江省首批名中医。此为 1933 年 12 月 4 日在杭州上城区上光华巷河下 10 号儿科诊所手书处方。

朱德明藏

Yi Zhiquan (1910-1977) was a renowned pediatrician in Hangzhou City. He was in the list of the first batch of Famous Chinese Medicine Practitioners of Zhejiang Province at the beginning of the founding of the People's Republic of China. This prescription was written by him at a Pediatric Clinic located at No.10 Guanghua Lane Shangcheng District, Hangzhou City.

Preserved by Zhu Deming

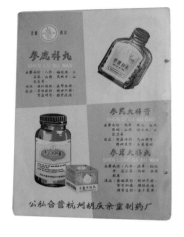

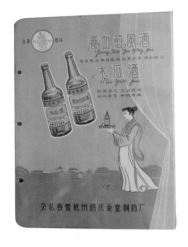

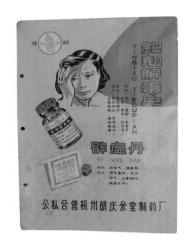

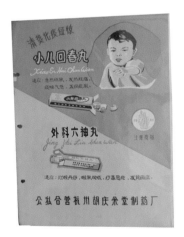

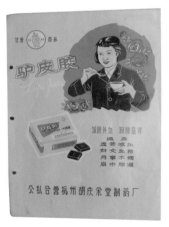

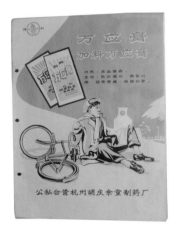

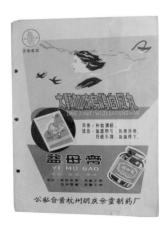

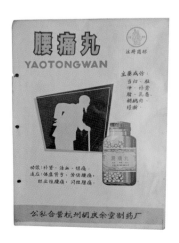

胡庆余堂制药厂广告

近现代

长 26.5 厘米，宽 19.5 厘米，一组 8 张

同治十三年 (1874 年) 一月，胡雪岩在杭州
直吉祥巷九头间设胡庆余堂雪记国药号筹备
处，光绪四年 (1878 年)，胡庆余堂大井巷
店屋落成开张。

朱德明藏

Advertising Posters of Hu Qing Yu Tang Pharmaceutical Factory

Modern Times

Length 26.5 cm/ Width 19.5 cm, 8 posters/set

In January of the 13th year of Emperor Tongzhi's Reign in the Qing Dynasty (1874), Hu Xueyan set up the preparatory office of Hu Qing Yu Tang (Xue's) Chinese Medicine Drugstore at Jiu Tou Jian, Zhi Ji Xiang Lane, Hangzhou City. In the 4th year of Emperor Guangxu's Reign (1878), Hu Qing Yu Tang (Dajing Lane Branch) was opened.

Preserved by Zhu Deming

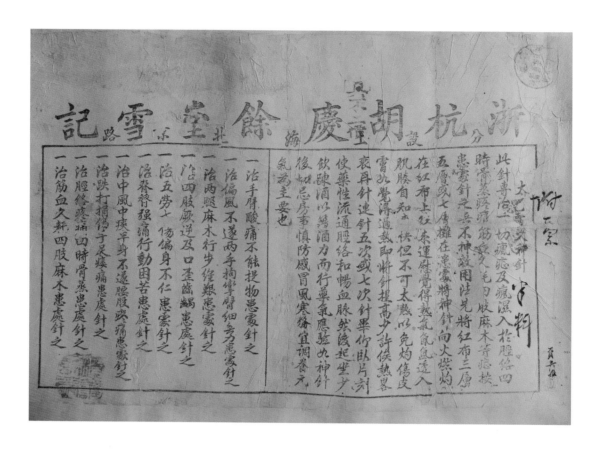

胡庆余堂太乙雷火神针仿单

近现代

长 40 厘米，宽 27 厘米

Instruction of Taiyi and Leihuo Needles of Hu Qing Yu Tang Drugstore

Modem Times

Length 40 cm/ Width 27 cm

同治十三年 (1874 年) 一月，胡雪岩在杭州
直吉祥巷九头间设胡庆余堂雪记国药号筹备
处，光绪四年 (1878 年)，胡庆余堂大井巷
店屋落成开张。

朱德明藏

In January of the 13th year of Emperor
Tongzhi's Reign in the Qing Dynasty (1874),
Hu Xueyan set up the preparatory office of
Hu Qing Yu Tang (Xue's) Chinese Medicine
Drugstore at Jiu Tou Jian, Zhi Ji Xiang Lane,
Hangzhou City. In the 4th year of Emperor
Guangxu's Reign (1878), Hu Qing Yu Tang
(Dajing Lane Branch) was opened.

Preserved by Zhu Deming

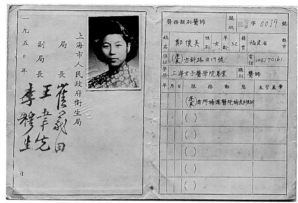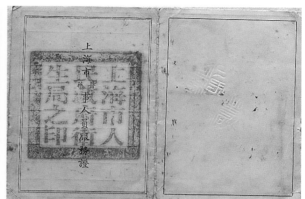

上海市医事人员服务证

近现代

10 厘米 ×8 厘米

Service Certificate of Shanghai Medical Personnel

Modem Times

10 cm×8 cm

我国妇产科学界老前辈,著名的妇产科专家,妇产科内分泌临床开创者之一,中华医学会妇产科学会生殖内分泌学组顾问郑怀美教授1950年《上海市医事人员服务证》。上海市人民政府卫生局崔义田局长签发。

上海医药文献博物馆藏

This Service Certificate of Shanghai Medical Personnel was issued in 1950 by Cui Yitian, director of Shanghai Health Bureau, for Professor Zheng Huaimei, a predecessor and expert in gynaecology and obstetrics, one of the endocrine clinical pioneers in gynecology and obstetrics, and consultant in the division of reproductive endocrinology, Society of Obstetrics and Gynecology, Chinese Medical Association.

Preserved in Shanghai Medical Literature Museum

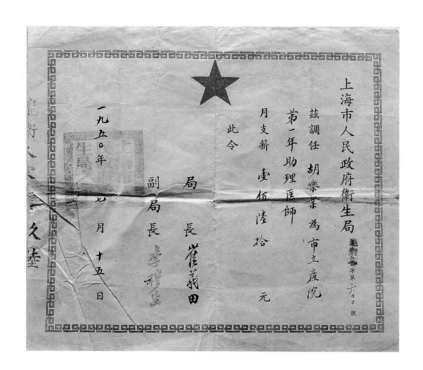

上海市立产院调令

近现代

25 厘米 ×20 厘米

Transfer Order for Shanghai Municipal Maternity Hospital

Modem Times

25 cm×20 cm

常识提醒我们：既然上海市第一妇婴保健院不叫"上海市妇婴保健院"，那应该还有"上海市第二妇婴保健院"。的确，云南曲靖市妇幼医院前身就是上海市第二妇婴保健院；而上海市第二妇婴保健院原名为上海市立产院。

上海医药文献博物馆藏

Common sense reminds us since Shanghai First Maternity and Infant Hospital is not called "Shanghai Maternity and Infant Hospital", there should be "Shanghai Second Maternity and Infant Hospital". Indeed, the predecessor of Yunnan Qujing Maternity and Child Health Hospital is Shanghai Second Maternity and Infant Hospital, which was formerly known as Shanghai Municipal Maternity Hospital.

Preserved in Shanghai Medical Literature Museum

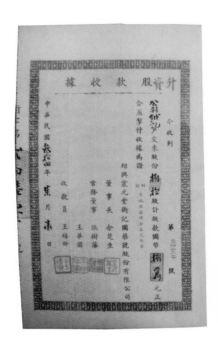 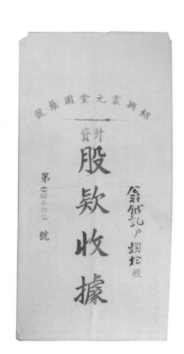

震元堂股票

近现代

左图：长 26 厘米，宽 16.5 厘米

右图：长 26 厘米，宽 11.3 厘米

Stock Certificate of Zhenyuan Tang

Modern Times

Left: Length 26 cm/ Width 16.5 cm

Right: Length 26 cm/ Width 11.3 cm

绍兴震元堂衡记国药号股份有限公司股票。震元堂初创于清乾隆十七年（1752），由杜景湘于城内水澄桥下开设。

朱德明藏

This was the stock certificate of Zhenyuan Tang Chinese Medicine Store Co., Ltd. Founded in 1752 during the reign of Emperor Qianlong of Qing Dynasty, Zhenyuan Tang was opened by Du Jingxiang under Shuicheng Bridge in the city.

Preserved by Zhu Deming

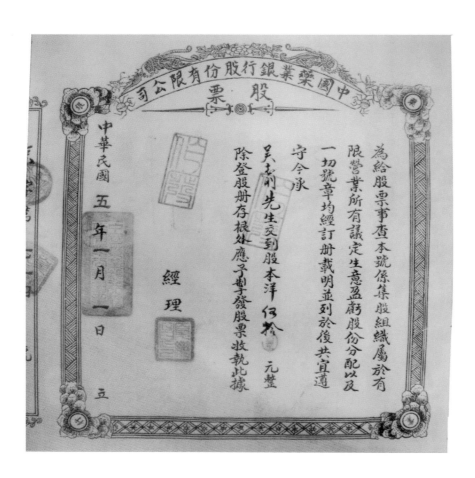

中国药业银行股份有限公司股票

近现代

长 26.5 厘米，宽 24.5 厘米

Stock Certificate of Pharmaceutical Bank of China Co., Ltd.

Modern Times

Length 26.5 cm/ Width 24.5 cm

吴志刚先生用大洋伍拾元整购买中国药业银行股份有限公司股票的凭证。

朱德明藏

This was the stock certificate of Pharmaceutical Bank of China Co., Ltd bought by Mr. Wu Zhigang with fifty silver dollars.
Preserved by Zhu Deming

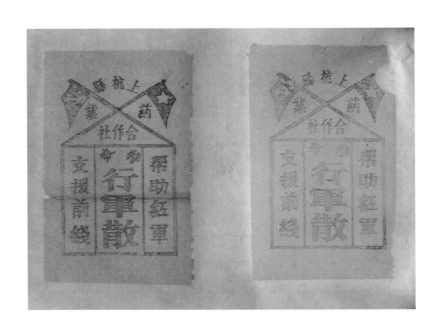

红军广告

民国

长 15 厘米，宽 9 厘米

江西省上杭县药业合作社特效"行军散"广告，帮助红军，支援前线。

朱德明藏

Advertisement of the Red Army

The Republic of China

Length15 cm/ Width 9 cm

This is an advertisement of specific "Xingjun Powder" produced by the Pharmaceutic Cooperation of Shanghang County, Jiangxi Province. It aimed at giving support to the Red Army and the frontline.

Preserved by Zhu Deming

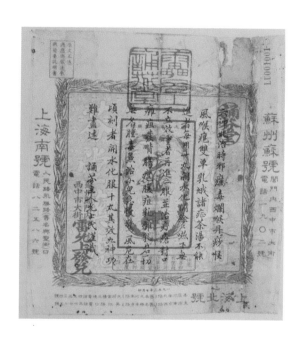

雷允上诵芬堂兑票

民国

长 20 厘米，宽 18 厘米

图为位于苏州阊门内西中市大街的雷允上诵芬堂六神丸兑票。

朱德明藏

Voucher of Lei Yunshang's Song Fen Tang Drugstore

The Republic of China

Length 20 cm/ Width 18 cm

The voucher was used to exchange for miraculous pills of six ingredients at Lei Yunshang's Song Fen Tang on Xizhongshi Street, Suzhou City.

Preserved by Zhu Deming

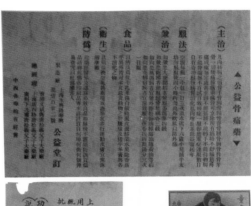

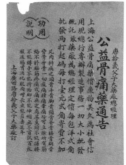

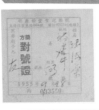
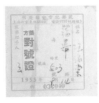
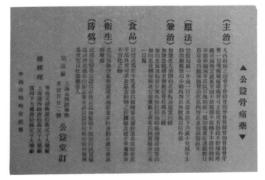
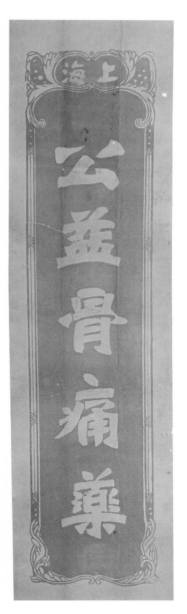

公益骨痛药广告

民国

长 57.5 厘米，宽 39 厘米

上海公益堂公益骨痛药广告。

朱德明藏

Advertisement of Gongyi Painkillers for Bone Pain

The Republic of China

Length 57.5 cm/ Width 39 cm

This is an advertisement of Gongyi Painkillers for Bone Pain by Shanghai Gongyi Tang Drugstore.

Preserved by Zhu Deming

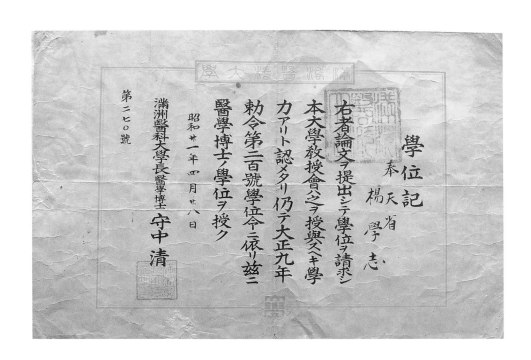

满洲医科大学学位证

民国

45 厘米 ×30 厘米

前江西省妇女保健院院长杨学志教授 1946 年满洲医科大学博士学位记——学位证。满洲医科大学为中国医科大学前身。

上海医药文献博物馆藏

Diploma of the Manchuria Medical University

The Republic of China

45 cm×30 cm

This doctorate certificate was awarded in 1946 to Yan Xuezhi. Professor Yan Xuezhi once was the director of the former Jiangxi Provincial Women's Health Care Center. Manchuria Medical University is now China Medical University.

Preserved in Shanghai Medical Literature Museum

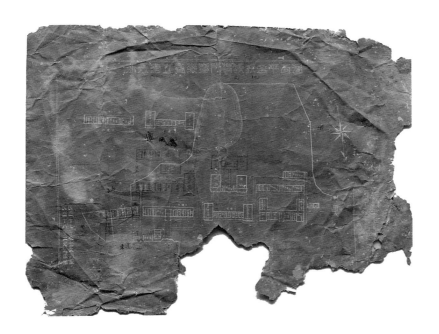

浙江省立医药专门学校校舍平面图

民国

60 厘米 ×40 厘米

浙江省立医药专门学校校舍平面图。1928 年俞哲文绘制，次年王克思重绘。浙江省立医药专门学校，今浙江大学医学院。

上海医药文献博物馆藏

Ichnography of Zhejiang Provincial Medical Specialized School

The Republic of China

60 cm×40 cm

The ichnography of Zhejiang Provincial Medical Specialized School was drawn by Yu Zhewen in 1928 and was redrawn by Wang Kesi in the following year. Zhejiang Provincial Medical Specialized School is now the School of Medicine, Zhejiang University.

Preserved in Shanghai Medical Literature Museum

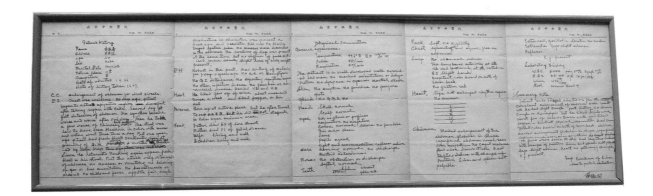

蒋福润医师住院病历

民国

25 厘米 ×20 厘米

南京中央医院蒋福润医师英文写就的住院病历。南京中央医院位于中山东路 205 号，现为南京军区南京总医院占用。该院是民国时期南京规模最大、设备最完善的国立医院。

上海医药文献博物馆藏

Medical Record by Dr. Jiang Furun

The Republic of China

25 cm×20 cm

It was a medical record written in English by Dr. Jiang Furun of Nanjing Central Hospital. The hospital was located at No.205 East Zhongshan Road, where is now Nanjing General Hospital of Nanjing Military Command. It was the biggest national hospital with the most complete facilities in Nanjing City during the Republican Period.

Preserved in Shanghai Medical Literature Museum

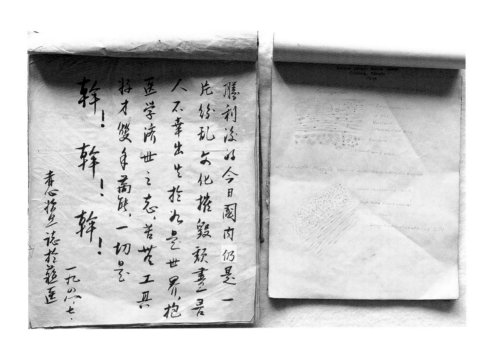

蒋鉴新教授笔记

民国

30 厘米 ×20 厘米

上海交通大学医学院已故蒋鉴新教授在国立江苏医学院读书时的《病理学》《解剖学》笔记。在其《解剖学》笔记的扉页，有这样一段话："抱医学济世之志……干！干！干！"

上海医药文献博物馆藏

Professor Jiang Jianxin's notes

The Republic of China

30 cm×20 cm

These are the notes of *Pathology* and *Anatomy* of professor Jiang Jianxin of the School of Medicine of Shanghai Jiaotong University when he was studying at National Jiangsu Medical College. On the flyleaf of his note of *Anatomy*, he wrote: "Learn Medicine to heal the world! Go! Go! Go!"

Preserved in Shanghai Medical Literature Museum

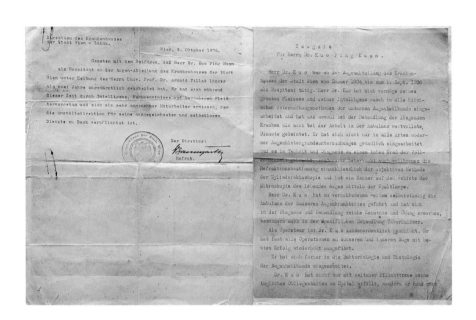

郭秉宽留学证明书

民国

30 厘米 ×20 厘米

1936 年，中国眼科之父郭秉宽教授从维也纳回国，图为奥地利医院院长为其出具的证明书。

上海医药文献博物馆藏

Guo Bingkuan's Study Abroad Certificate

The Republic of China

30 cm×20 cm

In 1936, the director of Austrian Hospital issued the certificate to Guo Bingkuan, the founding father of ophthalmology in China, before he came back to China from Vienna.

Preserved in Shanghai Medical Literature Museum Museum

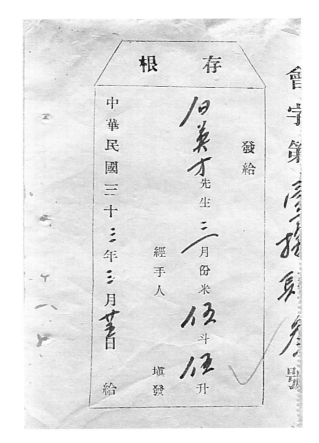

白英才收据

民国

18 厘米 ×15 厘米

1944 年 3 月，华西协和大学白英才教授"五斗五升"米收据。抗战期间，教授生活亦很艰难，有"五斗米教授"之说。

上海医药文献博物馆藏

Bai Yingcai's Receipt

The Republic of China

18 cm×15 cm

In March 1944, Pro. Bai Yingcai of Huaxi Medical University wrote the receipt of 5.5 "dou" rice. During the anti-Japanese war, even the professors lived a hard life. There was a saying like "Five-Dou （1 "dou"equals 10 liters） Rice Professor" to illustrate this.

Preserved in Shanghai Medical Literature Museum

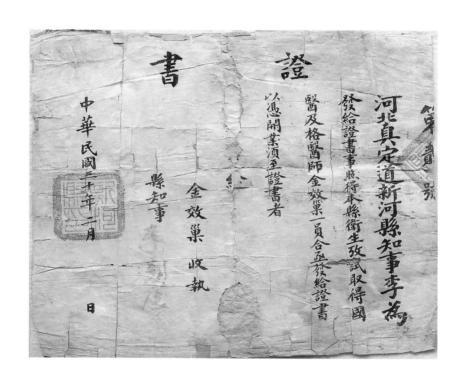

河北医师开业执照

民国

40 厘米 ×25 厘米

1941 年，河北真定道新河县知事李为颁发的开业执照，第 2 号。民国时期，县太爷多称"县长"，汪伪政权所辖区域称"知事"。

上海医药文献博物馆藏

Medical License in Hebei Province

The Republic of China

40 cm×25 cm

It was License No. 2 issued by "Zhishi" Li Wei of Xinhe County, Zhending District, Hebei Province. During the Republican period, the county magistrates were called "Xian Zhang", while in the areas under the jurisdiction of Wang's puppet regime, they were called "Zhishi".

Preserved in Shanghai Medical Literature Museum

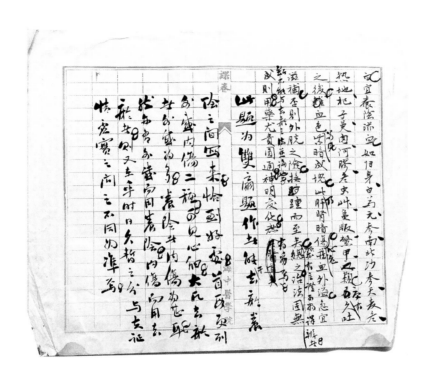

上海中医学院学生课卷

民国

40 厘米 ×25 厘米

民国时期上海中医学院学生课卷，有老师评语。

该校与今日的上海中医药大学不是传承关系。

上海医药文献博物馆藏

Student's Homework of Shanghai College of Chinese Medicine

The Republic of China

40 cm×25 cm

This is a student's written homework with teachers' comments in Shanghai College of Chinese Medicine, which has no relation with the present Shanghai College of Chinese Medicine.

Preserved in Shanghai Medical Literature Museum

Museum

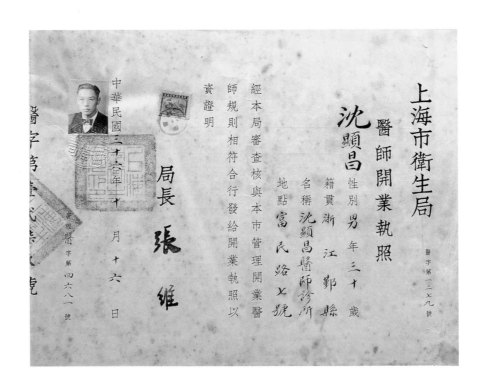

上海医师开业执照

民国

45 厘米 ×30 厘米

Medical License of Shanghai City

The Republic of China

45 cm×30 cm

1947 年 10 月，上海市卫生局局长张维为沈显昌医师签发的《医师开业执照》。

上海医药文献博物馆藏

In October 1947, the director of Shanghai Health Bureau, Zhang Wei, issued the License to Dr. Shen Xianchang.

Preserved in Shanghai Medical Literature Museum

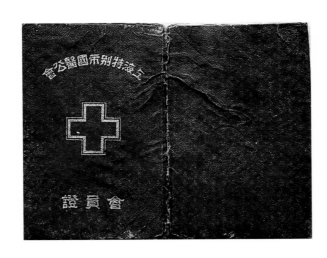
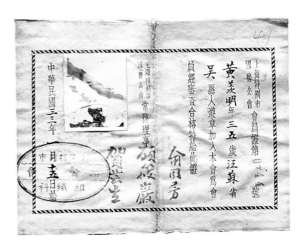

黄羡明《会员证》

民国

10 厘米 ×7 厘米

Membership Card

The Republic of China

10 cm×7 cm

上海特别市国医公会会员黄羡明的《会员证》。黄羡明，无锡人，历任上海市立第一人民医院针灸科主任兼上海中医学院针灸教研组副主任、上海市中医研究所副所长、上海市针灸经络研究所所长、中国上海国际针灸培训中心主任等。

上海医药文献博物馆藏

This card belonged to Huang Xianming, a member of Shanghai Chinese Medicine Association. Huang Xianming, born in Wuxi, served successively as the director of the Department of Acupuncture and Moxibustion of Shanghai Municipal First People's Hospital and the associate director of Acupuncture and Moxibustion Department of Shanghai Chinese Medical College, deputy director of Shanghai Research Institute of Traditional Chinese Medicine, director of Shanghai Institute of Acupuncture and Meridian, and the director of Shanghai International Acupuncture Training Center.

Preserved in Shanghai Medical Literature Museum

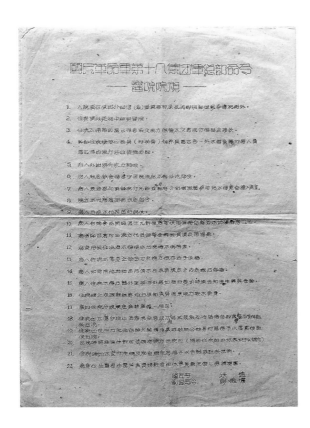

八路军医院院规

民国

35 厘米 ×25 厘米

红色文献——《国民革命军第十八集团军医院院规》。总司令：朱德；副总司令：彭德怀。

上海医药文献博物馆藏

Regulations of Eight Route Army Hospitals

The Republic of China

35 cm×25 cm

This is literature of Red Revolution—Regulations of the Eighteenth Army Hospital of the National Revolutionary Army. Commander In Chief: Zhu De. Deputy Commander In Chief: Peng Dehuai.

Preserved in Shanghai Medical Literature Museum

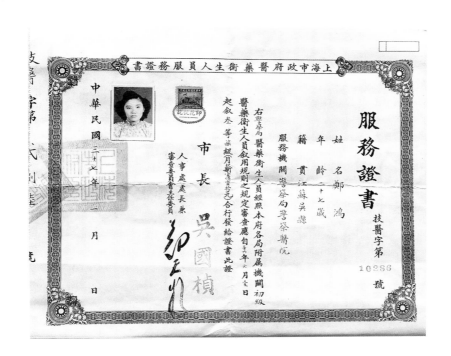

医务人员服务证书

民国

45 厘米 ×30 厘米

1948 年 1 月，民国上海市最后一任市长吴国桢
为警察局警察医院医务人员签发的《服务证书》。
警察局警察医院，今上海市中西医结合医院。

上海医药文献博物馆藏

Certificate of Medical Service

The Republic of China

45 cm×30 cm

In January 1948, Wu Guozhen, the last mayor of
Shanghai during Republican Period issued the
certificate of service for medical staffs of the Police
Hospital of Shanghai Police Office. Police Hospital
of Shanghai Police Office is now Integrated Chinese
and Western Medicine Hospital.

Preserved in Shanghai Medical Literature Museum

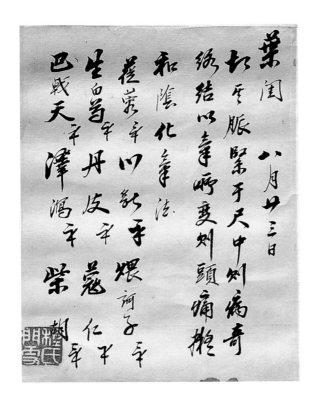

程门雪处方笺

民国

30 厘米 ×25 厘米

程门雪处方。1954 年，程门雪出任上海市第
十一人民医院（今上海曙光医院）中医科主任。
1956 年，上海中医学院创建，程门雪任该院首
任院长。

上海医药文献博物馆藏

Cheng Menxue's Prescription

The Republic of China

30 cm×25 cm

This prescription was written by Cheng Menxue,
who was appointed as the director of the Traditional
Chinese Medicine Department of Shanghai Eleventh
People's Hospital (now as Shanghai Shuguang
Hospital) in 1954, and as the first president of
Shanghai College of Traditional Chinese medicine.
Preserved in Shanghai Medical Literature Museum
Museum

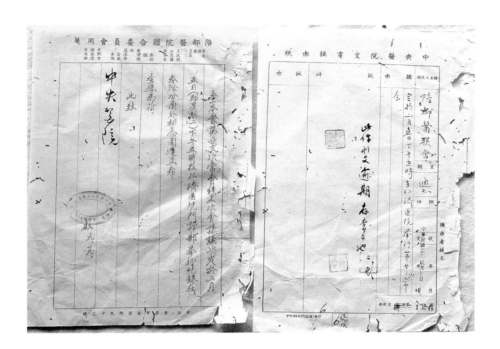

陪都医院联合委员会用笺

民国

30 厘米 ×25 厘米

陪都医院联合委员会用笺。陪都，指重庆。陪都
医院联合委员会委员：沈克菲、胡兰生、朱恒璧、
陈崇寿、锐朴、梁正伦、刘启承、甘怀杰。

上海医药文献博物馆藏

Document Paper of the Joint Committee of Peidu Hospital

The Republic of China

30cm×25cm

This is the document paper used by the Joint Committee of Peidu Hospital. Peidu refers to Chongqing. Members of the Joint Committee of Peidu Hospital are: Shen Kefei, Hu Lansheng, Zhu Hengbi, Chen Chongshou, Rui Pu, Liang Zhenglun, Liu Qicheng, and Gan Huaijie.

Preserved in Shanghai Medical Literature Museum Museum

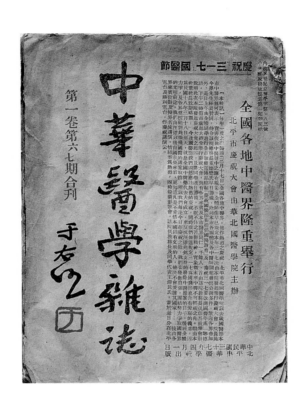

中医界创办的《中华医学杂志》

民国

30 厘米 ×25 厘米

中国医学史上，同时存在过两本《中华医学杂志》，一本由中华医学会主办，本图为另一本由北平中华医学社主办。

上海医药文献博物馆藏

Chinese Medical Journal by CMA

The Republic of China

30 cm×25 cm

In the history of Chinese medicine, there existed two versions of *Chinese Medical Journal*: one was founded by Chinese Medical Association (CMA) and the other shown in this picture was founded by Peking Chinese Medical Society.

Preserved in Shanghai Medical Literature Museum

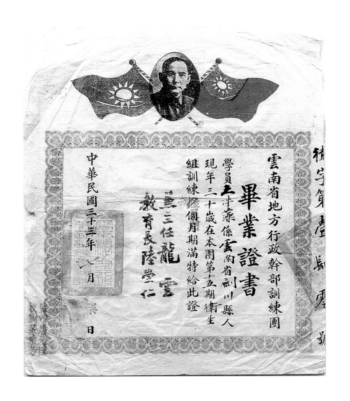

云南省地方行政干部训练团毕业证书

民国

35 厘米 ×25 厘米

1944 年，云南省地方行政干部训练团卫生组学员毕业证书。训练团主任：龙云；教育长：陆学仁。

上海医药文献博物馆藏

Training Certificate of Yunnan Provincial Administrators

The Republic of China

35 m×25 cm

This is the certificate for members of the Medical Training Corps. Director of the Training Corps: Long Yun. Head of Education: Lu Xueren.

Preserved in Shanghai Medical Literature Museum

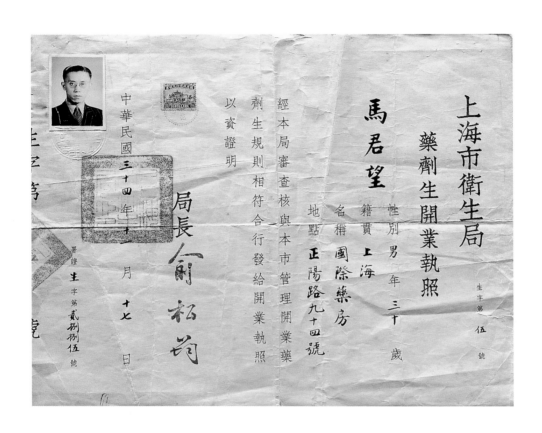

《**药剂生开业执照**》

民国

45 厘米 ×35 厘米

License for Pharmacist

The Republic of China

45 cm×35 cm

1945 年，上海市卫生局局长俞松筠为马君望药剂师签发的《药剂生开业执照》。俞松筠（1898—1951），陈果夫外甥。1922 年创建私立中德医院（黄浦区妇幼保健院），自任院长，后任上海中德高级助产职业学校校长。1945 年 8 月 20 日至 1946 年 5 月任上海特别市卫生局局长。

上海医药文献博物馆藏

It was issued to pharmacist Ma Junwang by Yu Songyun, director of Shanghai Health Bureau, in 1945. Yu Songyun (1898-1951) is the nephew of Chen Guofu. In 1922, he founded Private Sino-German Hospital (Huangpu Maternity and Child Health Care Center) and was self-appointed as the director. Later, he was the president of Shanghai Sino-Germen Advanced Midwifery Vocational School. From August 20, 1945 to May 1946, he was the director of Shanghai Health Bureau.

Preserved in Shanghai Medical Literature Museum

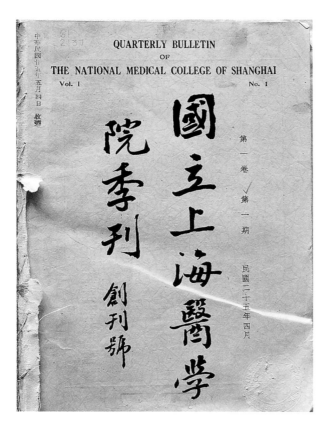

《国立上海医学院季刊》

民国

35 厘米 ×25 厘米

1936 年《国立上海医学院季刊》创刊号。

上海医药文献博物馆藏

Quarterly Bulletin of the National Medical College of Shanghai

The Republic of China

35 cm×25 cm

This is the commencing issue of *Quarterly Bulletin of the National Medical College of Shanghai* in 1936.

Preserved in Shanghai Medical Literature Museum

《震旦医刊》

民国

35 厘米 ×25 厘米

1938 年《震旦医刊》。1948 年，王振义院士从震旦大学医学院毕业，获得医学博士学位，因成绩优异，留在广慈医院（瑞金医院）担任住院医师。

上海医药文献博物馆藏

Bulletin Medical de L'universite L'aurore

The Republic of China

35 cm ×25 cm

This is an issue of *Bulletin Medical de L'universite L'aurore* published in 1938. In 1948, the academician Wang Zhenyi graduated from Medical College of Shanghai and received his doctorate. Because of his outstanding performance, he was employed as the resident doctor at Guangci Hospital (today's Ruijin Hospital).

Preserved in Shanghai Medical Literature Museum

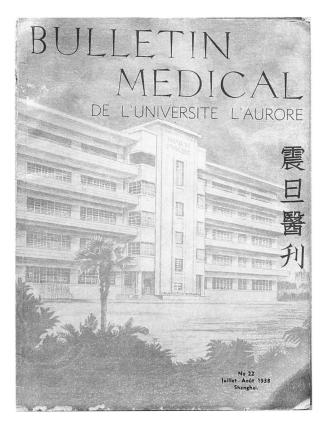

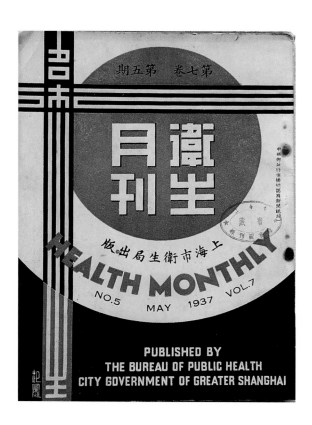

《卫生月刊》

民国

35 厘米 ×25 厘米

1937 年上海市卫生局出版的《卫生月刊》。

上海医药文献博物馆藏

Health Monthly

The Republic of China

35 cm ×25 cm

Health Monthly was published by the Bureau of Public Health City Government of Shanghai in 1937.

Preserved in Shanghai Medical Literature Museum

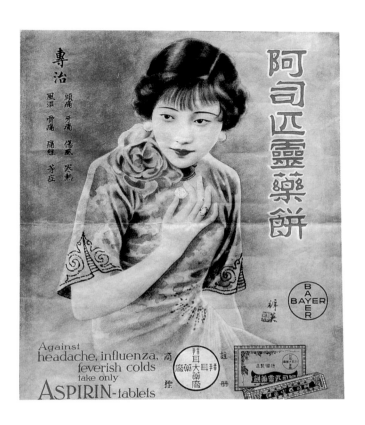

阿司匹林药饼广告

民国

60 厘米 ×40 厘米

德国拜耳阿司匹林药饼广告。杭穉英作品。平面
模特：阮玲玉。

上海医药文献博物馆藏

Advertisement of Aspirin Tablets

The Republic of China

60 cm ×40 cm

This is an advertisement poster of German Bayer's
aspirin tablets, designed by Hang Zhiying. The
model on it is Ruan Lingyu.

Preserved in Shanghai Medical Literature Museum

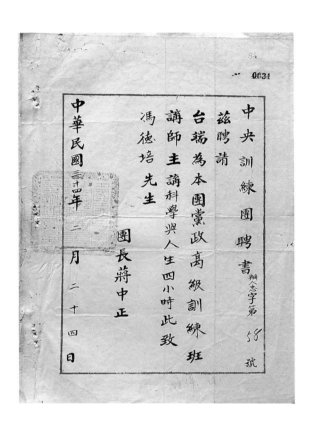

中央训练团聘书

民国

20 厘米 ×16 厘米

Appointment Letter of Central Training Corps

The Republic of China

20 cm ×16 cm

1945 年，蒋介石为冯德培教授签发的《中央训练团聘书》。冯德培于 1926 年毕业于复旦大学生物学院。1934 年起，历任北京协和医学院、北京师范大学讲师、副教授；1943 年，任上海医学院教授；1981 年 5 月，任中国科学院副院长。1995 年逝世。

上海医药文献博物馆藏

This is the letter of appointment signed by Jiang Jieshi to Professor Feng Depei in 1945. In 1926, Feng graduated from College of Biological Sciences of Fudan University. From 1934, Feng successively worked at Peking Union Medical College as a lecturer and Beijing Normal University as an associate professor. Then in 1943, Feng became the professor in Medical College of Shanghai. In May 1981, Feng was selected as vice-president of the Chinese Academy of Sciences.

Preserved in Shanghai Medical Literature Museum

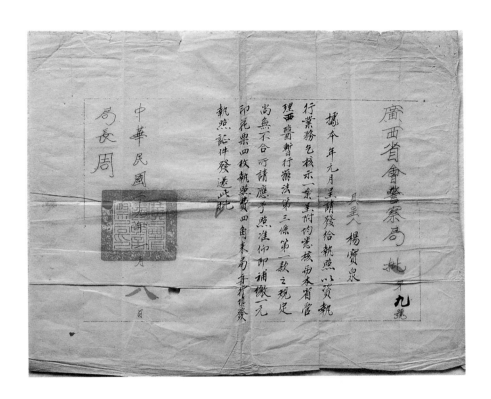

广西医师执照

民国

60 厘米 ×40 厘米

Guangxi Provincial Medical License

The Republic of China

60 cm×40 cm

1940 年，广西省会警察局给杨宝泉医师的执照批示。民国时期，警察局权限很宽、权力极大。

上海医药文献博物馆藏

This is Doctor Yang Baoquan's medical license instructed by Guangxi provincial police office in 1940. During the Republican period (1912–1949), police office had wide administration range and high authority.

Preserved in Shanghai Medical Literature Museum

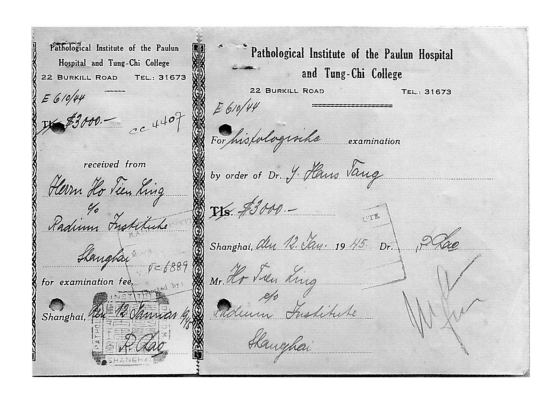

病理报告单

民国

20 cm×15 cm

Pathological Report

The Republic of China

20 cm×15 cm

1945 年，上海同济大学医学院附属宝隆医院病理研究所出具的病理报告。宝隆医院由德国医生宝隆 1900 年创建于上海，1955 年迁至武汉。现附属于华中科技大学同济医学院。

上海医药文献博物馆藏

In 1945, the pathological report was provided by the Institute of Pathology of Paulun Hospital affiliated to Tongji University School of Medicine, Shanghai. Paulun Hospital was founded by German doctor Paulun in Shanghai in 1900 and then moved to Wuhan in 1955. Now it is affiliated to Tongji Medical College of Huazhong University of Science and Technology (HUST).

Preserved in Shanghai Medical Literature Museum

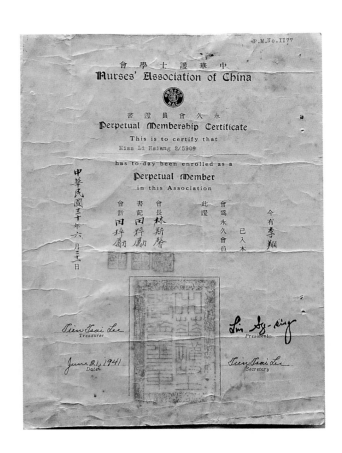

中华护士学会会员证

民国

30 厘米 ×22 厘米

Membership Certificate of Nurses' Association of China

The Republic of China

30 cm×22 cm

1941年，中华护士学会为李翔小姐签发的《永久会员证书》。当时，会长为护理学家林斯馨先生。

上海医药文献博物馆藏

In 1941, the Nurses' Association of China issued this Perpetual Membership Certificate to Miss. Li Xiang. At that time, the president of the Association was Mr. Lin Sixin, a nursing expert.

Preserved in Shanghai Medical Literature Museum

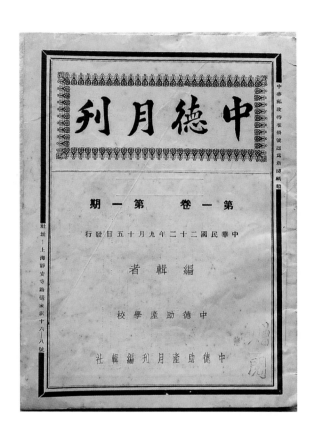

《中德月刊》

民国

30 厘米 ×25 厘米

Sino-German Monthly

The Republic of China

30 cm×25 cm

1933 年 9 月，《中德月刊》创刊号。中德医院，
今上海市黄埔区妇幼保健院。

上海医药文献博物馆藏

This is the commencing issue of *Sino-German
Monthly* in September, 1933. Sino-German
Hospital is now the Maternity and Child Health
Hospital of Shanghai Huangpu District.
Preserved in Shanghai Medical Literature
Museum

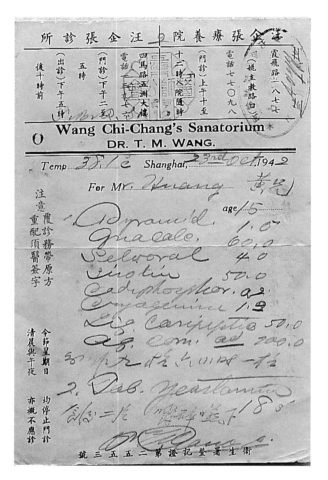

汪企张处方

民国

15 厘米 ×10 厘米

Prescription Written by Wang Qizhang

The Republic of China

15 cm×10 cm

1942 年，汪企张处方。在 1928 年全日教育
会议上，汪企张首次提出废止中医案，未获
通过。

上海医药文献博物馆藏

The prescription was written by Wang Qizhang
in 1942. In 1928, Wang Qizhang first proposed
the abolition of Chinese medicine at the full-
time education conference, but his proposal was
not approved.

Preserved in Shanghai Medical Literature
Museum

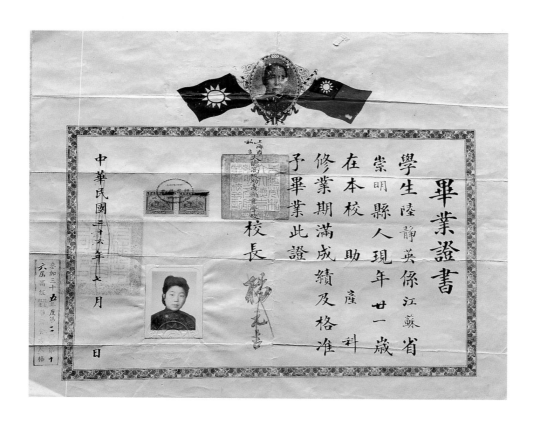

上海市私立大德高级助产职业学校毕业证

民国

45 厘米 ×30 厘米

Shanghai Dade Senior Midwifery Vocational School Diploma

The Republic of China

45 cm×30 cm

江苏省崇明县人陆静英上海市私立大德高级
助产职业学校毕业证，校长杨元吉。大德助
产学校与上海市第一妇婴保健院渊源颇深。
杨元吉是我国妇产科学奠基人之一。

上海医药文献博物馆藏

The diploma belongs to Lu Jingying, a native
of Chongming County, Jiangsu Province. The
president of the school at that time was Yang
Jiyuan, one of the founders of Chinese sciences
of obstetrics and gynecology. Dade Senior
Midwifery Vocational School and Shanghai
First Maternity and Infant Hospital are
profoundly related.
Preserved in Shanghai Medical Literature
Museum

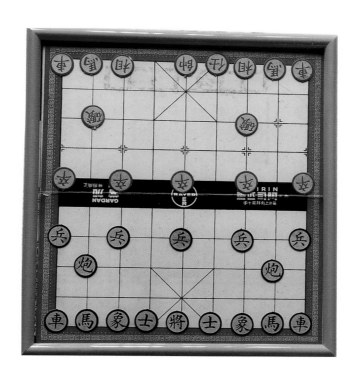

象棋棋盘与棋子

民国

25 厘米 ×25 厘米

拜耳药厂象棋棋盘与棋子——早期的产品提示物。注意"礮"字。

上海医药文献博物馆藏

Board and Pieces of Chinese Chess

The Republic of China

25 cm×25 cm

The board and pieces of Chinese Chess have the logo of a pharmaceutical enterprise called Bayer. This was one of the brand awareness tools at the early time. The Chinese character " 礮 " is the original complex form of " 炮 " (cannon).

Preserved in Shanghai Medical Literature Museum

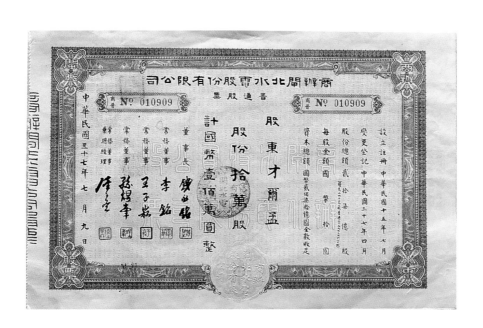

闸北水电股份有限公司股票

民国

25 厘米 ×20 厘米

1948 年闸北水电股份有限公司股票，股东才尔孟。才尔孟 1947—1949 年间任广慈医院院长；1949 为常务校董；1951 年被驱逐出境。

上海医药文献博物馆藏

Stock Certificate of Zhabei Hydropower Co., Ltd.

The Republic of China

25 cm×20 cm

This was the stock certificate of Zhabei Hydropower Co., Ltd. in 1948. The stockholder was Germain (French) who worked as the president of Sainte-Marie Hospital in 1947–1949 and the manager of the board of trustees in 1949, and who was deported from China in 1951.

Preserved in Shanghai Medical Literature Museum

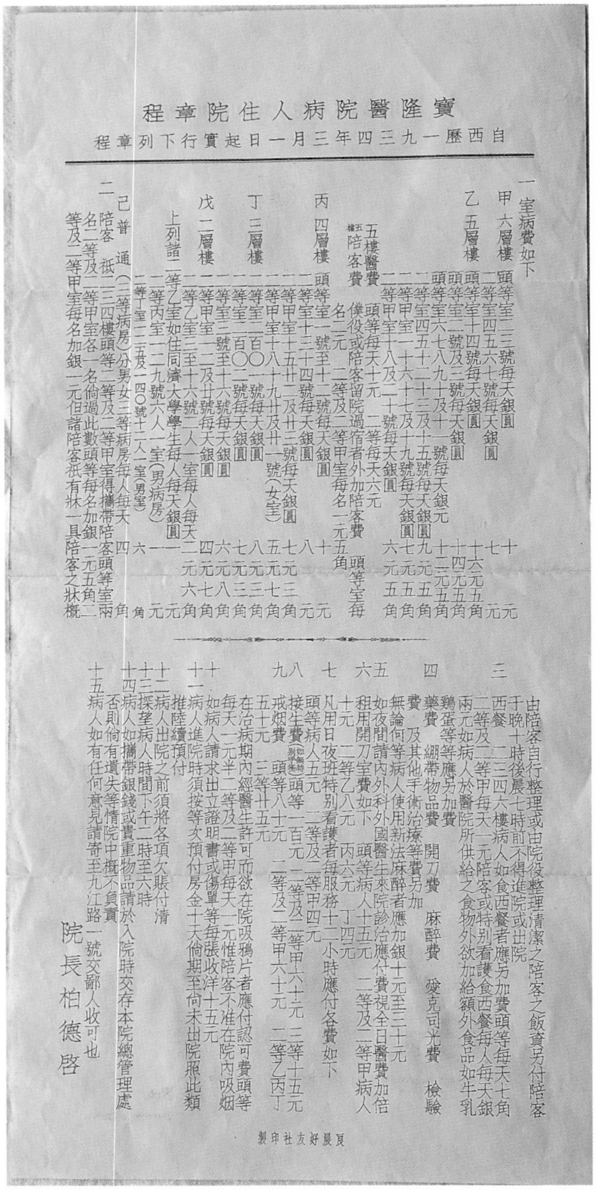

寶隆醫院病人住院章程

自西歷一九三四年三月一日起實行下列章程

一 室病費如下

甲 六層樓 頭等室二三號每天銀圓 十元

二等室四五六七號每天銀圓 七元

乙 五層樓 頭等室十四號每天銀圓 十六元五角

頭等室二號及三號每天銀圓 十四元五角

頭等室六七八九十及十一號每天銀元 十二元五角

二等室四五十二十三及十五號每天銀圓 九元五角

二等甲室一十六十七及十九號每天銀圓 七元五角

二等甲室十八及二十號每天銀圓 六元五角

五樓醫費 頭等每天十元 二等每天六元

（五樓）陪客費 僕役或陪客留院過宿者外加陪客費頭等室每名二元 二等及二等甲室每名一元五角

丙 四層樓 頭等室一號至十二號每天銀圓 十元

二等室十三十四號每天銀圓 八元

二等甲室十五廿二及廿三號每天銀圓 七元三角

二等甲室十八十九廿及廿一號（女室）每天銀圓 五元七角

丁 三層樓 二等室二百〇一號每天銀圓 八元三角

二等室二百〇二號每天銀圓 七元三角

二等室三號至十六號每天銀圓 六元八角

戊 二層樓 二等甲室一二及廿號每天銀圓 四元七角

二等乙室三至十六號二人一室每人每天 二元六角

上列諸二等乙室如住同濟大學學生每人每天銀圓 一元

二等丙室一二九號六人一室（男病房） 一元

二等丁室一二五及一四〇號十二人一室（男室） 六角

己 普通（三等病房）分男女三等病房每人每天 四角

二 陪客 祗二三四樓頭等二等及二等甲室得攜帶陪客頭等室兩名二等及二等甲室各一名倘過此數頭等每名加銀一元五角二等及二等甲室每名加銀一元但諸陪客祗有牀一具陪客之牀概由陪客自行整理或由院役整理清潔之陪客之飯資另付陪客

三 于晚十時後晨七時前不得進院或出院

西餐 二三四六樓病人如食西餐者應另加費頭等每天七角 二等及二等甲每天一元陪客或特別看護食西餐每人每天銀兩元如病人於醫院所供給之食物外欲加給額外食品如牛乳鷄蛋等等應另加費

四 藥費 綳帶物品費 開刀費 麻醉費 愛克司光費 檢驗費及其他手術治療等費另加

無論何等病人使用新法麻醉者應加銀十元至三十元

如夜間請內外科外國醫生來院診治應付費視全日醫費加倍

五 租用開刀室費如下 頭等病人十五元 二等及二等甲病人十元 二等乙八元 丙六元 丁四元

六 凡用日夜班特別看護者每服務十二小時應付各費如下 頭等病人五元 二等及二等甲四元

七 接生費（如無特別手術）頭等一百元 二等及二等甲六十元 三等十五元

八 戒烟費 頭等八十元 二等及二等甲六十元 二等乙丙丁五十元 三等廿五元

九 在治病期內經醫生許可而欲在院吸鴉片者應付認可費頭等每天一元半二等及二等甲每天一元惟陪客不准在院內吸烟

十 如病人請求出立證明書或傷單等每張收洋十五元

十一 病人進院時須按等次預付房金十天倘期至尚未出院照此類推陸續預付

十二 病人出院之前須將各項欠賬付清

十三 探望病人時間下午二時至六時

十四 病人如攜帶銀錢或貴重物品請於入院時交存本院總管理處否則倘有遺失等情院中概不負責

十五 病人如有任何意見請寄至九江路一號交鄙人收可也

院長柏德啓

良晨好友社印製

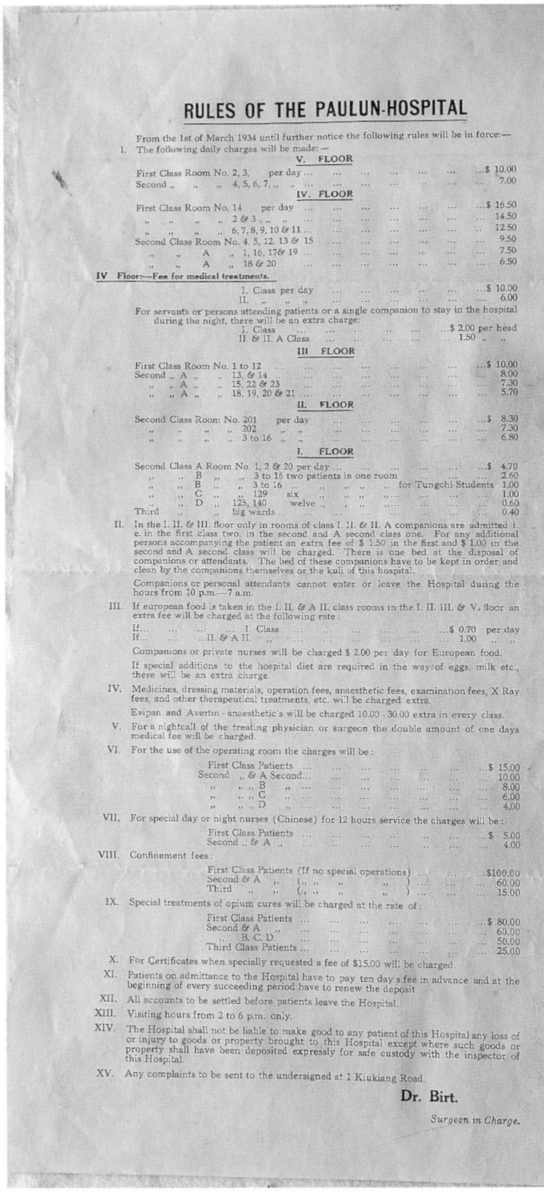

RULES OF THE PAULUN-HOSPITAL

From the 1st of March 1934 until further notice the following rules will be in force:—

I. The following daily charges will be made: —

V. FLOOR

First Class Room No. 2, 3, per day ... ...$ 10.00
Second „ „ „ 4, 5, 6, 7, „ „ ... 7.00

IV. FLOOR

First Class Room No. 14 per day ... ...$ 16.50
„ „ „ „ 2 & 3 „ „ ... 14.50
„ „ „ „ 6, 7, 8, 9, 10 & 11 ... 12.50
Second Class Room No. 4, 5, 12, 13 & 15 ... 9.50
„ „ A „ 1, 16, 17& 19 ... 7.50
„ „ A „ 18 & 20 ... 6.50

IV Floor:—Fee for medical treatments.

I. Class per day ... ...$ 10.00
II. „ „ „ ... 6.00

For servants or persons attending patients or a single companion to stay in the hospital during the night, there will be an extra charge:

I. Class ... ...$ 2.00 per head
II. & II. A Class ... 1.50 „ „

III FLOOR

First Class Room No. 1 to 12 ... ...$ 10.00
Second „ A „ „ 13, & 14 ... 8.00
„ „ A „ „ 15, 22 & 23 ... 7.30
„ „ A „ „ 18, 19, 20 & 21 ... 5.70

II. FLOOR

Second Class Room No. 201 per day ... ...$ 8.30
„ „ „ „ 202 „ „ ... 7.30
„ „ „ „ 3 to 16 „ „ ... 6.80

I. FLOOR

Second Class A Room No. 1, 2 & 20 per day ... ...$ 4.70
„ „ B „ „ 3 to 16 two patients in one room ... 2.60
„ „ B „ „ 3 to 16 „ „ „ „ „ for Tungchi Students 1.00
„ „ C „ „ 129 six „ „ „ „ ... 1.00
„ „ D „ 125, 140 welve „ „ „ „ ... 0.60
Third „ „ big wards... ... 0.40

II. In the I. II. & III. floor only in rooms of class I. II. & II. A companions are admitted i. e. in the first class two, in the second and A second class one. For any additional persons accompanying the patient an extra fee of $ 1.50 in the first and $ 1.00 in the second and A second class will be charged. There is one bed at the disposal of companions or attendants. The bed of these companions have to be kept in order and clean by the companions themselves or the kuli of this hospital.

Companions or personal attendants cannot enter or leave the Hospital during the hours from 10 p.m.—7 a.m.

III. If european food is taken in the I. II. & A II. class rooms in the I. II. III. & V. floor an extra fee will be charged at the following rate:

If... ... ... I. Class ... ...$ 0.70 per day
If... ... ...II. & A II. „ ... 1.00 „ „

Companions or private nurses will be charged $ 2.00 per day for European food.

If special additions to the hospital diet are required in the way of eggs, milk etc., there will be an extra charge.

IV. Medicines, dressing materials, operation fees, anaesthetic fees, examination fees, X Ray fees, and other therapeutical treatments, etc. will be charged extra.

Evipan and Avertin - anaesthetic's will be charged 10.00 - 30.00 extra in every class.

V. For a nightcall of the treating physician or surgeon the double amount of one days medical fee will be charged.

VI. For the use of the operating room the charges will be:

First Class Patients ... ...$ 15.00
Second „ & A Second... ... 10.00
„ „ „ B „ ... 8.00
„ „ „ C „ ... 6.00
„ „ „ D „ ... 4.00

VII. For special day or night nurses (Chinese) for 12 hours service the charges will be:

First Class Patients ... ...$ 5.00
Second „ & A „ ... 4.00

VIII. Confinement fees:

First Class Patients (If no special operations) $100.00
Second & A „ („ „ „ „) ... 60.00
Third „ „ („ „ „ „) ... 15.00

IX. Special treatments of opium cures will be charged at the rate of:

First Class Patients ... ...$ 80.00
Second & A „ ... 60.00
„ B. C. D. „ ... 50.00
Third Class Patients 25.00

X. For Certificates when specially requested a fee of $15.00 will be charged.

XI. Patients on admittance to the Hospital have to pay ten day's fee in advance and at the beginning of every succeeding period have to renew the deposit

XII. All accounts to be settled before patients leave the Hospital.

XIII. Visiting hours from 2 to 6 p.m. only.

XIV. The Hospital shall not be liable to make good to any patient of this Hospital any loss of or injury to goods or property brought to this Hospital except where such goods or property shall have been deposited expressly for safe custody with the inspector of this Hospital.

XV. Any complaints to be sent to the undersigned at 1 Kiukiang Road.

Dr. Birt.

Surgeon in Charge.

宝隆医院住院章程

民国

50 厘米 ×20 厘米

1934 年宝隆医院住院章程。病室分甲、乙、丙、丁、戊、己六等，日住院费从 10 元到 4 角不等，可以满足不同阶层的医疗需求。宝隆医院迁至武汉以后，旧址为上海长征医院所占。

上海医药文献博物馆藏

Rules of Paulun Hospital

The Republic of China

50 cm×20 cm

In 1934, Paulun Hospital carried out these rules, according to which the wards were ranked from A to F with daily hospitalization expenses ranging from 10 yuan to 0.4 yuan so as to meet the medical needs of different classes. After Paulun Hospital was moved to Wuhan City, its original site was occupied by Shanghai Changzheng Hospital.

Preserved in Shanghai Medical Literature Museum

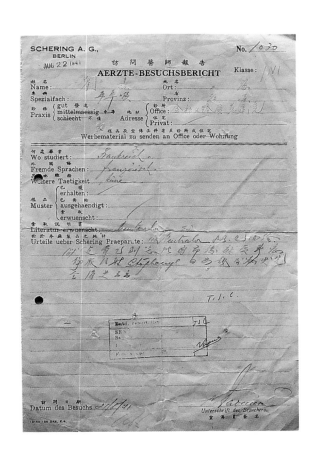

《访问医师报告》

民国

25 厘米 ×20 厘米

Physician Visiting Report

The Republic of China

25 cm ×20 cm

这是笔者所看到的最早的《访问医师报告》，即《医药代表拜访日志》，填写于 1941 年。该报告由德国先灵的"宣传员"，即医药代表填写。被访医院广慈，今瑞金也。被访医生刘焘为知名五官科专家。

上海医药文献博物馆藏

Physician Visiting Report, namely, Log of Medical Representative's Visit, is the earliest report the author has ever seen. The report was filled by a medical representative concurrently one of promoters of German Schering A. G. in 1941. The visited hospital was Guangci Hospital, known as Ruijin hospital today. The visited doctor is Liu Tao, a famous expert in ophthalmology and otorhinolaryngology.

Preserved in Shanghai Medical Literature Museum

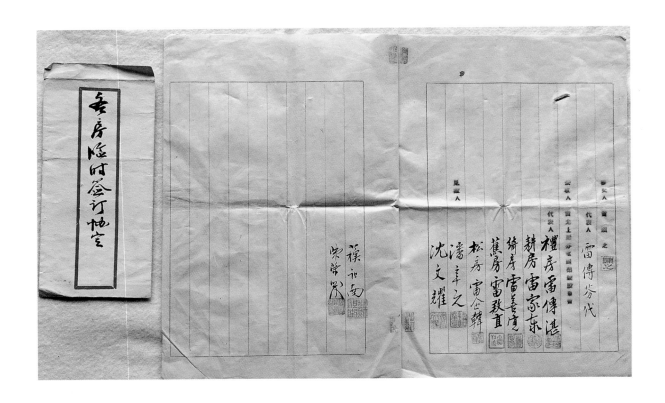

雷允上协议

民国

40 厘米 ×30 厘米

Agreement of Lei Yunshang Drugstore

The Republic of China

40 cm ×30 cm

民国末年，雷允上《各房临时签定协定》。
当时，雷家分五房：礼房、耕房、绮房、蕉房、
松房。

上海医药文献博物馆藏

This is the Temporary Agreement of Lei
Yunshang's offsprings signed in the end of the
Republic Period. At that time, Lei family had
five subdivisions: Li, Geng, Qi, Jiao, and Song.
Preserved in Shanghai Medical Literature Museum

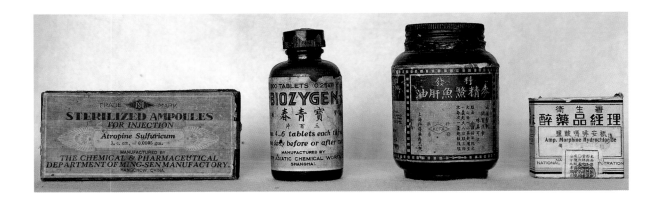

药瓶、药盒一组

民国

纸、玻璃等

5~15 厘米

Medicine Packages and Bottles

The Republic of China

Paper and Glass

5-15 cm

杭州民生阿托品、上海新亚宝青春、上海科发鱼肝油、卫生署盐酸吗啡之药盒。郑筱萸局长曾任杭州民生制药厂厂长。科发，建于1909年，由德国医生科发 (Dr.Kuifuss) 创办。

上海医药文献博物馆藏

These are packages and bottles of the following medicines respectively: Atropine Sulfuricum produced by the Chemical &Pharmaceutical Department of Ming-sen Manufactory, Biozygen by New Asiatic Chemical Works, Cod Liver Oil by Kefa Pharmaceutical Manufactory and Amp. Morphine Hydrochloride by Department of Health. The former general director of National Food and Drug Administration, Zheng Xiaoyu, was once appointed as the head of the Chemical & Pharmaceutical Department of Ming-sen Manufactory of Hangzhou City. Kefa Pharmaceutical Manufactory was established by German Dr. Kuifuss in 1909.

Preserved in Shanghai Medical Literature Museum

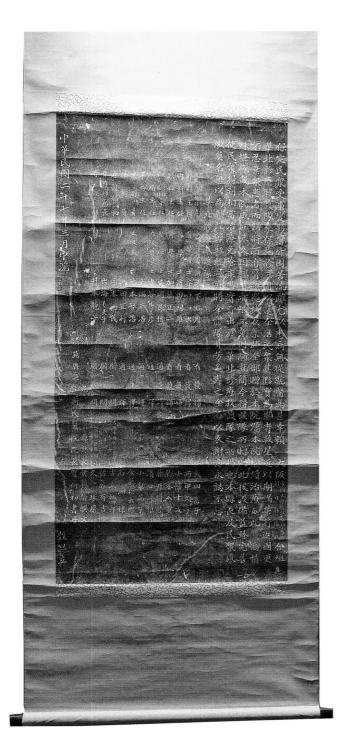

清苑县立新民医院拓片

民国

120 厘米×60 厘米

Rubbing of Qingyuan Prefectural Xinmin Hospital

The Republic of China

120 cm×60 cm

1938 年，日本华北诊疗救护队在保定诊疗三个月，临行将所有医疗器械及药品赠予清苑县立新民医院等。从拓片的裱工看，此物属于日本回流。

上海医药文献博物馆藏

In 1938, the Japanese first-aid team for diagnosis and treatment worked in North China for 3 months. Before leaving, the team donated all the medical equipment and drugs to Qingyuan prefectural Xinmin hospital and other hospitals. Judging from the mounting of the rubbing, the author thinks that it was spread from Japan.

Preserved in Shanghai Medical Literature Museum

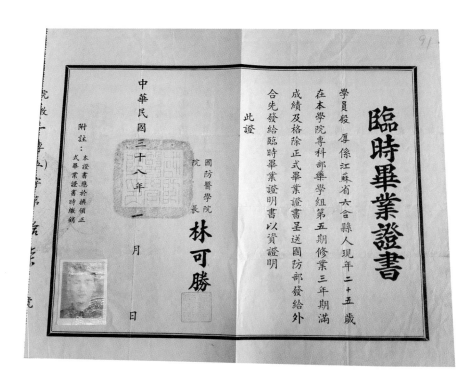

国防医学院临时毕业证

民国

45 厘米 × 30 厘米

Temporary Diploma of National Defense Medical Center (NDMC)

The Republic of China

45 cm×30 cm

1949 年 1 月国防医学院临时毕业证。院长：林可胜中将。国防医学院，或称国防医学中心，简称国医，创立于 1902 年，是中华民国时期军事院校中历史最悠久之学府。现址位于我国台北市内湖区。直属教学医院为台北市三军总医院。

上海医药文献博物馆藏

This is the temporary diploma of National Defense Medical Center in January 1949. Its president was lieutenant general Lin Kesheng. National Defense Medical Center, shortly known as NDMC, was founded in 1902. It enjoys the longest history among all military colleges in the Republic of China (1912-1949). The site is now located in the Neihu District of Taipei of China. The teaching hospital Directly under the jurisdiction of NDMC is Tri-Service General Hospital of Taipei of China.

Preserved in Shanghai Medical Literature Museum

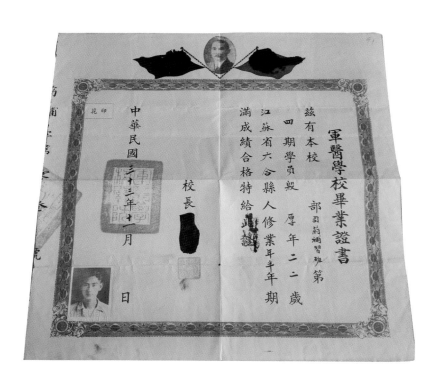

军医学校毕业证

民国

45 厘米×30 厘米

1944 年军医学校毕业证，校长蒋中正。1944 年的军医学校位于贵州安顺。该校为国防医学院前身。

上海医药文献博物馆藏

Diploma of Military Medical School

The Republic of China

45 cm×30 cm

This is the diploma of military medical school in 1944, located in Anshun City, Guizhou Province. The president was Jiang Zhongzheng. This school was the predecessor of National Defense Medical Center.

Preserved in Shanghai Medical Literature Museum

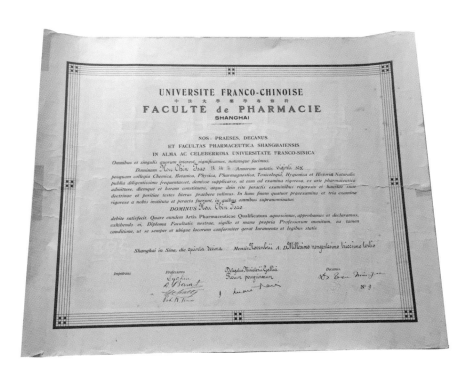

中法大学毕业证

民国

55 厘米×45 厘米

上海中法大学药学专修科毕业证。该校后来并入复旦大学医学院。顾学裘教授毕业于该校。

上海医药文献博物馆藏

Diploma of China-France University

The Republic of China

55 cm×45 cm

This is the diploma of Pharmacy Junior College of Shanghai China-France University. The school was later merged into Medical School of Fudan University. Professor Gu Xueqiu also graduated from the School.

Preserved in Shanghai Medical Literature Museum

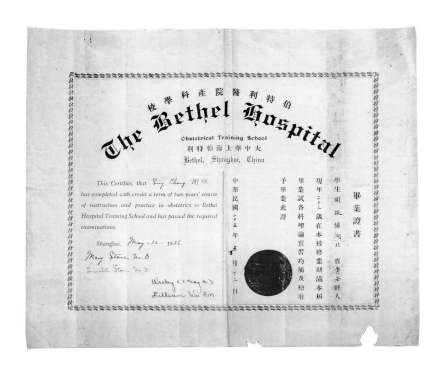

伯特利医院毕业证

民国

45 厘米×35 厘米

Diploma of the Bethel Hospital

The Republic of China

45 cm×35 cm

上海市第九人民医院前身——伯特利医院附属产科学校毕业证。此证于 1936 年 5 月由 Mary stone——石美玉颁发给谢振同学。

上海医药文献博物馆藏

This is the diploma of Affiliated Obstetrical Training School of the Bethel Hospital, which was the predecessor of Shanghai Ninth People's Hospital. The diploma was awarded by Ms. Mary Stone (Chinese name Shi Meiyu) to a student named Xie Zhen in May 1936.

Preserved in Shanghai Medical Literature Museum

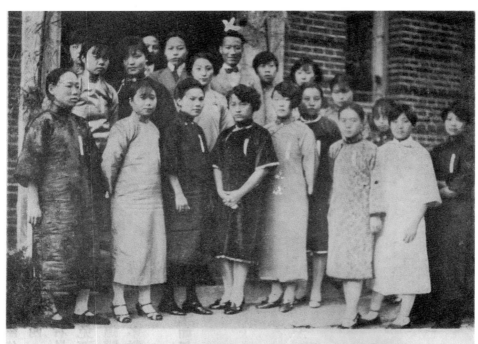

大華產科醫校開幕之時招待之中有X者
即校長金變章（岑衡慶攝）

民国残报

民国

30 厘米×20 厘米

Incomplete newspaper of the Republic of China (1912-1949)

The Republic of China

30 cm×20 cm

这张照片来自一份民国残报。大华产科医校为大华医院附属学校。校长和院长均为金燮章医师。1926 年，西医掀起一种风气，以大华医院为名，聘请各科专家，门诊一次要收费一百银元。其实当时有许多公立医院，门诊费不超过一元、二元，住院也不过八元、十元。

上海医药文献博物馆藏

This photo shows a piece of incomplete newspaper of the Republic of China (1912–1949). Dahua Obstetric Medical School was affiliated to Dahua Hospital. The president of the hospital and school is physician Jin Xiezhang. In 1926, there was a phenomenon in western medicine field that experts of different departments were engaged under the name of Dahua Hospital, charging a hundred silver dollars for outpatients each time. In fact, many public hospitals just charged no more than one or two silver dollars for outpatients and no more than eight to ten silver dollars for hospitalization at that time.

Preserved in Shanghai Medical Literature Museum

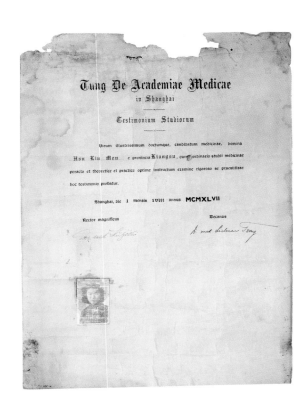

同德医学院毕业证书

民国

55 厘米×35 厘米

Diploma of Tung De Medical School

The Republic of China

55 cm×35 cm

《同德医学院毕业证书》

苏林梦女士，来自江苏省，完成了医学课程，且以杰出的优异的的成绩，通过了严格的理论和最佳的实践操作考试。

特此颁发证书

上海　　　1947 年 7 月 1 日

院长　　　xxx

上海医药文献博物馆藏

In the Diploma of Tung De Medical School, it writes in German that: This is to certificate that Ms Su Linmeng from Jiangsu Province accomplished her medical courses and got a very excellent result through both strict theories and the best practice exams.

There is the signature of the Dean's name. The date was on July 1st, 1947.

Preserved in Shanghai Medical Literature Museum

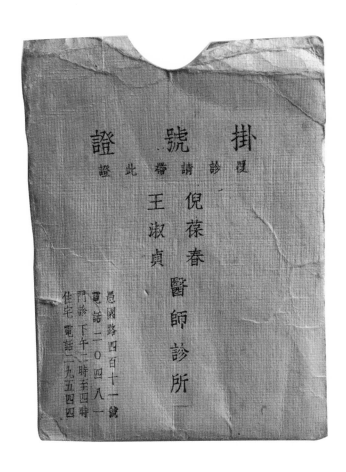

挂号证袋

民国

10 厘米×7 厘米

Bag for Register Card

The Republic of China

10 cm×7 cm

王淑贞、倪葆春为医界伉俪。王淑贞是我国
妇产科泰斗，红房子医院院长。倪葆春教授
是我国整形外科之父，1936 年即在上海圣约
翰大学医学院附属同仁医院建立国内第一个
整形外科。

上海医药文献博物馆藏

The names on the cover were a couple in the
field of medicine. Zhang Shuzhen, the leading
expert in obstetrics and gynecology in China,
was the president of Shanghai Red House
Hospital. Professor Ni Baochun is the father
of plastic surgery in China. In 1936, the first
Orthopedics Hospital was established by him
in Tongren Hospital affiliated to School of
Medicine, St. John's University, Shanghai.
Preserved in Shanghai Medical Literature
Museum

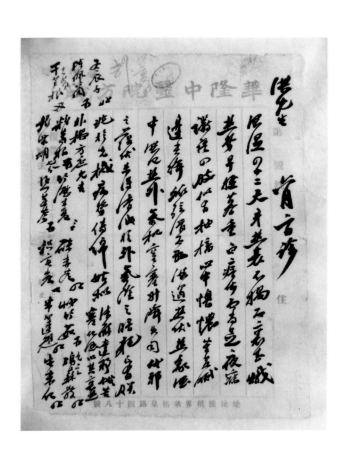

华隆中医院方笺

民国

长 28 厘米，宽 20.5 厘米

图为位于上海法租界华格泉路 48 号的华隆中医院方笺。

朱德明藏

Hualong Chinese Medicine Hospital's Prescription

The Republic of China

Length 28 cm/ Width 20.5 cm

This hospital was located at No. 48 Huagequan Road French Concession District, Shanghai city.

Preserved by Zhu Deming

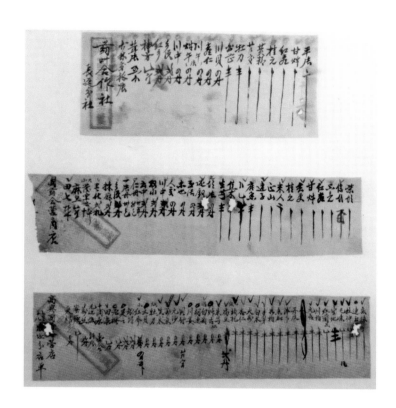

红军处方

民国

上：长 13 厘米，宽 13.5 厘米

中：长 41.5 厘米，宽 10.5 厘米

下：长 42 厘米，宽 11 厘米

中国工农红军第一后方医院药叶合作社长迳分社处方。

朱德明藏

Prescriptions for the Red Army

The Republic of China

Upper: Length 30 cm/ Width 13.5 cm

Middle: Length 41.5 cm/ Width 10.5 cm

Lower: Length 42 cm/ Width 11 cm

The prescriptions were given by Changjing branch of Pharmaceutical Cooperative of the No.1 Military Rear Hospital of the Chinese Workers' and Peasants' Red Army.

Preserved by Zhu Deming

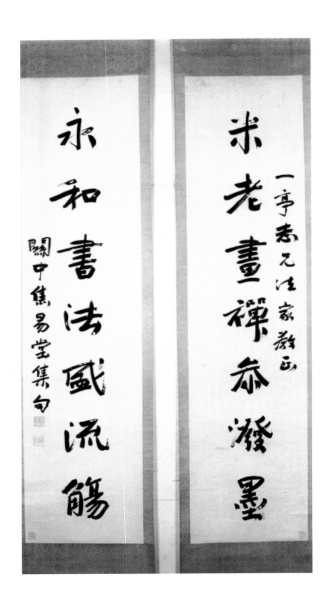

焦易堂书联

民国

长 161 厘米，宽 38 厘米

焦易堂，被孙中山誉为"秦中杰士"，1929 年任国民政府法制委员会委员长，在中医废存大战中力挺中医。1937 年 3 月 17 日任中央国医馆馆长。

上海中医药博物馆藏

Couplets Written by Jiao Yitang

The Republic of China

Length 161 cm/ Width 38 cm

Jiao Yitang, praised by Sun Yat-sen as "A Great Person from Shaanxi", was appointed as the Chairman of the National Government Legal Committee. He firmly supported the traditional Chinese medicine during the disputation of whether to reserve or abolish it, and then he became the director of Central Traditional Chinese Medicine Center in March 17, 1937. Preserved in Shanghai Museum of Traditional Chinese Medicine

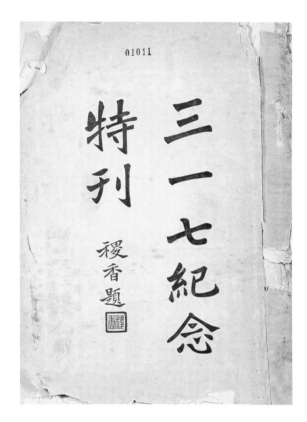

《三一七纪念特刊》

民国

27.1 厘米 × 19.5 厘米

1929 年 3 月 17 日，全国中医药界发起抗议国民政府废止中医案活动，并取得成功，为此发行纪念特刊。

上海中医药博物馆藏

Special Issue for Memorializing Event on March 17

The Periods of the Republic of China

27.1 cm×19.5 cm

On March 17, 1929, national Chinese medicine industry started an activity to protest the government for its bill to abolish Traditional Chinese Medicine, and they won. So the special issue was to commemorate this.

Preserved in Shanghai Museum of Traditional Chinese Medicine

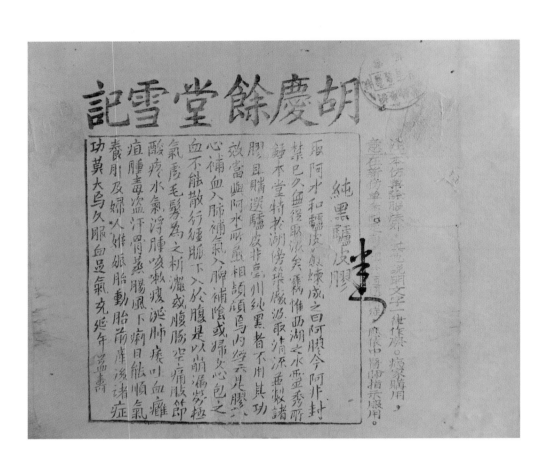

胡庆余堂纯黑驴皮胶仿单

民国

长 23 厘米，宽 21 厘米

Instruction of Black Donkey-hide Gelatin

The Republic of China

Length 23 cm/ Width 21 cm

同治十三年（1874 年）一月，胡雪岩在杭州直吉祥巷九头间设胡庆余堂雪记国药号筹备处，光绪四年（1878 年），胡庆余堂大井巷店屋落成开张。

朱德明藏

In January of the 13th year of Emperor Tongzhi's Reign in the Qing Dynasty (1874), Hu Xueyan set up the preparatory office of Hu Qing Yu Tang (Xue's) Chinese Medicine Drugstore at Jiu Tou Jian, Zhi Ji Xiang Lane, Hangzhou City. In the 4th year of Emperor Guangxu's Reign (1878), Hu Qing Yu Tang (Dajing Lane Branch) was opened.

Preserved by Zhu Deming

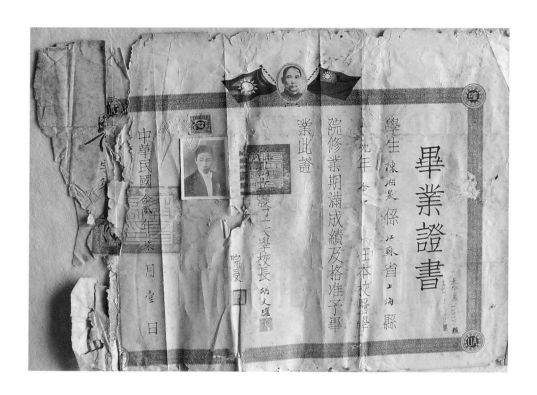

陈湘泉教授毕业证

民国

60 厘米×45 厘米

Diploma of Professor Chen Xiangquan

The Republic of China

60 cm×45 cm

陈湘泉，1933 年毕业于上海私立震旦大学医学院。曾任中国防痨协会上海分会总干事。1950 年岁末任广慈医院董事长。广慈，今上海瑞金医院。

上海医药文献博物馆藏

Chen Xiangquan graduated from the Medical College of Aurora University in 1933. He was the general director of Shanghai Branch of Chinese Antituberculosis Association. At the end of 1950, he was appointed as the president of Guangci Hospital, which is now Shanghai Rui Jin Hospital.

Preserved in Shanghai Medical Literature Museum

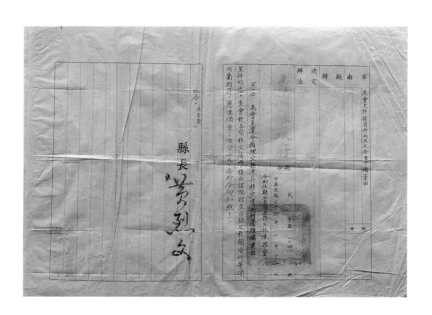

青浦县县立医院文书

民国

50 厘米×35 厘米

民国 34 年，青浦县县长黄烈文给县立医院医务主任朱振声的指令。

上海医药文献博物馆藏

Official Dispatch of Qingpu County Hospital

The Republic of China

50 cm×35 cm

It was the dispatch order for Zhu Zhensheng, medical officer of the hospital, released by Huang Liewen, county magistrate of Qingpu County.

Preserved in Shanghai Medical Literature Museum

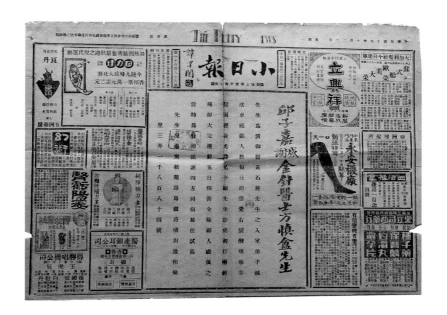

《小日报》

民国

60 厘米 ×50 厘米

1930 年 10 月 21 日的《小日报》，头版刊登大幅广告——邱子嘉感谢金针医士方慎盦先生。

上海医药文献博物馆藏

The Petty News

The republic of China

60 cm×50 cm

The newspaper was issued on October 21, 1930. On the front page was an advertisement entitled "Gratitude from Qiu Zijia to Acupuncturist Fang Shen'an".

Preserved in Shanghai Medical Literature Museum

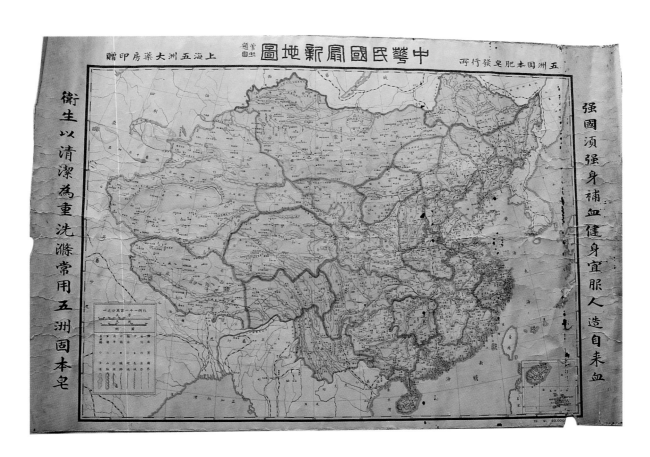

《中华民国新地图》

New Atlas of Republican China

民国

70 厘米 ×55 厘米

1929 年印制的《中华民国新地图》，由上海五洲大药房印赠。

上海医药文献博物馆藏

The Republic of China

70 cm×55 cm

The atlas was printed in 1929 and donated by Shanghai Continental Grand Pharmacy.

Preserved in Shanghai Medical Literature Museum

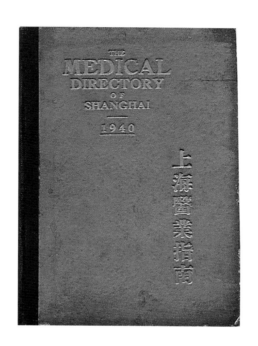

《上海医业指南》

民国

20 厘米×15 厘米

1940 年出版的《上海医业指南》，内有上海医院、医师、牙医的海量信息。

上海医药文献博物馆藏

Manual of Shanghai Medical Industry

The Republic of China

20 cm×15 cm

Issued in 1940, this manual contains massive information about hospitals, doctors and dentists in Shanghai.

Preserved in Shanghai Medical Literature Museum

索　引

（馆藏地按拼音字母排序）

上海中医药博物馆

Index

Shanghai Museum of Traditional Chinese Medicine

532

参考文献

[1] 李经纬 . 中国古代医史图录 [M]. 北京：人民卫生出版社，1992.

[2] 傅维康，李经纬，林昭庚 . 中国医学通史：文物图谱卷 [M]. 北京：人民卫生出版社，2000.

[3] 和中浚，吴鸿洲 . 中华医学文物图集 [M]. 成都：四川人民出版社，2001.

[4] 上海中医药博物馆 . 上海中医药博物馆馆藏珍品 [M]. 上海：上海科学技术出版社，2013.

[5] 西藏自治区博物馆 . 西藏博物馆 [M]. 北京：五洲传播出版社，2005.

[6] 崔乐泉 . 中国古代体育文物图录：中英文本 [M]. 北京：中华书局，2000.

[7] 张金明，陆雪春 . 中国古铜镜鉴赏图录 [M]. 北京：中国民族摄影艺术出版社，2002.

[8] 文物精华编辑委会员 . 文物精华 [M]. 北京：文物出版社，1964.

[9] 谭维四 . 湖北出土文物精华 [M]. 武汉：湖北教育出版社，2001.

[10] 常州市博物馆 . 常州文物精华 [M]. 北京：文物出版社，1998.

[11] 镇江博物馆 . 镇江文物精华 [M]. 合肥：黄山书社，1997.

[12] 贵州省文化厅，贵州省博物馆 . 贵州文物精华 [M]. 贵阳：贵州人民出版社，2005.

[13] 徐良玉 . 扬州馆藏文物精华 [M]. 南京：江苏古籍出版社，2001.

[14] 昭陵博物馆，陕西历史博物馆 . 昭陵文物精华 [M]. 西安：陕西人民美术出版社，1991.

[15] 南通博物苑 . 南通博物苑文物精华 [M]. 北京：文物出版社，2005.

[16] 邯郸市文物研究所 . 邯郸文物精华 [M]. 北京：文物出版社，2005.

[17] 张秀生，刘友恒，聂连顺，等 . 中国河北正定文物精华 [M]. 北京：文化艺术出版社，1998.

[18] 陕西省咸阳市文物局 . 咸阳文物精华 [M]. 北京：文物出版社，2002.

[19] 安阳市文物管理局 . 安阳文物精华 [M]. 北京：文物出版社，2004.

[20] 深圳市博物馆 . 深圳市博物馆文物精华 [M]. 北京：文物出版社，1998.

[21]《中国文物精华》编辑委员会 . 中国文物精华（1993）[M]. 北京：文物出版社，1993.

[22] 夏路，刘永生 . 山西省博物馆馆藏文物精华 [M]. 太原：山西人民出版社，1999.

[23] 文物精华编辑委员会 . 文物精华 [M]. 北京：文物出版社，1957.

[24] 山西博物院，湖北省博物馆 . 荆楚长歌：九连墩楚墓出土文物精华 [M]. 太原：山西人民出版社，2011.

[25] 刘广堂，石金鸣，宋建忠 . 晋国雄风：山西出土两周文物精华 [M]. 沈阳：万卷出版公司，2009.

[26] 沈君山，王国平，单迎红 . 滦平博物馆馆藏文物精华 [M]. 北京：中国文联出版社，2012.

[27] 张家口市博物馆 . 张家口市博物馆馆藏文物精华 [M]. 北京：科学出版社，2011.

[28] 浙江省文物考古研究所 . 浙江考古精华 [M]. 北京：文物出版社，1999.

[29] 故宫博物院 . 故宫雕刻珍萃 [M]. 北京：紫禁城出版社，2004.

[30] 故宫博物院紫禁城出版社 . 故宫博物院藏宝录 [M]. 上海：上海文艺出版社，1986.

[31] 首都博物馆 . 大元三都 [M]. 北京：科学出版社，2016.

[32] 新疆维吾尔自治区博物馆 . 新疆出土文物 [M]. 北京：文物出版社，1975.

[33] 王兴伊，段逸山 . 新疆出土涉医文书辑校 [M]. 上海：上海科学技术出版社，2016.

[34] 刘学春 . 刍议医药卫生文物的概念与分类标准 [J]. 中华中医药杂志，2016，31（11）:4406-4409.

[35] 上海古籍出版社 . 中国艺海 [M]. 上海：上海古籍出版社，1994.

[36] 紫都，岳鑫 . 一生必知的 200 件国宝 [M]. 呼和浩特：远方出版社，2005.

[37] 谭维四 . 湖北出土文物精华 [M]. 武汉：湖北教育出版社，2001.

[38] 张建青 . 青海彩陶收藏与鉴赏 [M]. 北京：中国文史出版社，2007.

[39] 银景琦 . 仫佬族文物 [M]. 南宁：广西人民出版社，2014.

[40] 廖果，梁峻，李经纬 . 东西方医学的反思与前瞻 [M]. 北京：中医古籍出版社，2002.

[41] 梁峻，张志斌，廖果，等 . 中华医药文明史集论 [M]. 北京：中医古籍出版社，2003.

[42] 郑蓉，庄乾竹，刘聪，等 . 中国医药文化遗产考论 [M]. 北京：中医古籍出版社，2005.